THE NEW-ENGLAND FARRIER;
OR, A
COMPENDIUM OF FARRIERY
IN FOUR PARTS

By Paul Jewett, Of Rowley

New Edition, With Valuable Additions

Exeter:
Published By Josiah Richardson

· · · · · · · · · · · · · · · · · · · ·

1826

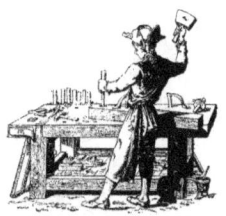

The Toolemera Press

www.toolemerabooks.com

The New-England Farrier; Or, A Compendium Of Farriery, In Four Parts
By Paul Jewett, Of Rowley
Exeter: Published by Josiah Richardson
1826

No part of this book may be reproduced, stored in an electronic retrieval system, or transmitted in any form or by an means, electronic, mechanical, photocopy, photographic or otherwise without the written permission of the publisher.

Excerpts of one page or less for the purposes of review and comment are permissible.

Copyright © 2013 The Toolemera Press
All rights reserved.

International Standard Book Number
ISBN : 978-0-9897477-6-9
(Trade Paper)

Published by
The Toolemera Press
Massachusetts U.S.A.

Manufactured in the United States of America

www.toolemerabooks.com

Introduction

The New England Farrier, by Paul Jewett of Rowley, Massachusetts, was first published in 1795 by William Barrett of Newburyport, Massachusetts. Subsequent editions by other publishers were printed in 1807, 1810, 1821, 1822, 1826, 1828, 1835 and 1840.

That first edition of 1795 gives *The New England Farrier* the honor of being the first book of farriery to have been both authored and published entirely within the continental United States of America.

Before the advent of the formal profession of the Veterinarian, the Farrier, who saw to the care of the hooves of horses, cows and other hoofed animals, was also called upon to treat the general ills that might befall the livestock of the farm. Even after towns and cities acquired the services of a Veterinarian, the Farrier, while engaged in providing care to the hooves of his patients, would often be called upon to offer up remedies and advice based upon both tradition and experience.

In many rural localities, the Farrier might also serve as the lone provider of medical advice to the farmer and family. Thus, *The New England Farrier* includes sections devoted to remedies for the ills that might befall adults and children who had little access to formal medical care.

Biography - Paul Jewett

The Jewett family of Rowley, Massachusetts has a long history, amongst which are a number of whom bear the first name of 'Paul'. The most likely candidate as author of *The New England Farrier* is:

Paul Jewett; Born March 13, 1739 - Rowley, County of Essex, Province Of Massachusetts Bay (one of the original thirteen states if the United States, later to become The Commonwealth Of Massachusetts); Died August 29, 1828 - Rowley, MA.

The Revolutionary War Rolls of The State Of Massachusetts provide the information that in Captain Silas Adams' Company of Colonel Asa Whitcomb's Regiment, dated November 29, 1776, one Paul Jewett of Rowley, MA served as a Private. Additional service records indicate that Paul Jewett enlisted on at least three separate occasions of at two months each, for a total of six months during the time period of 1776-1777.

Book Owner Signature - John & Alice Drew

This original copy was owned and signed by John J. Drew of Barrington, New Hampshire, 18??; Alice Drew, Barrington, New Hampshire, 1830; and again by John J. Drew, Barrington, New Hampshire, 1836.

John Drew was born in Barrington, New Hampshire, on April 11, 1811. He married Alice Waterhouse and had eleven children. He passed away in 1850.

Toolemera Reprints
www.toolemerabooks.com

- The Military Exercise Of The Independent Company of Cadets: Boston 1816

- The Little Confectioner: Smith Hicks 1876

- Text Book Of Swedish Home Sloyd: Anna P. Berg 1925

- The Teacher's Hand-Book Of Slojd: Otto Salomon 1892

- Mechanick Exercises: Joseph Moxon 1703

- The Mechanic's Companion: Peter Nicholson 1850

- The Student's Instructor In Drawing And Working The Five Orders Of Architecture: Peter Nicholson 1815

- The Circle Of The Mechanical Arts: Thomas Martin 1813

- The Complete Cabinet-Maker's And Upholsterer's Guide: J. Stokes 1829

- A Manual Of Wood Carving: Charles G. Leland, Revised by John J. Holtzapffel 1891

- Wood Carving: Joseph Phillips 1896

- Woodwork Tools And How To Use Them: William Fairham 1922

- Woodwork Joints: William Fairham 1920

- Cabinet Construction: J. C. S. Brough 1930

- Furniture Making: Advanced Projects In Woodwork: Ira Griffith 1912
- The Painter, Gilder, And Varnisher's Companion: H. C. Baird 1850
- Our Workshop: Temple Thorold 1866
- Carpentry And Joinery For Amateurs: James Lukin 1879
- The Art Of Mitring: Owen Maginnis 1892
- Working Drawings Of Colonial Furniture: F. Bryant 1922

The Toolemera Press reprints classic books, photographs and ephemera on early crafts, trades and industries, all carefully selected from our personal library.

www.toolemerabooks.com

Mr. John T. Drew
Barrington
N. H.
1852

THE

NEW-ENGLAND FARRIER;

OR, A

COMPENDIUM OF FARRIERY,

IN FOUR PARTS:

Wherein most of the Diseases to which Horses, Neat Cattle, Sheep and Swine are incident, are treated of; with Medical and Surgical observations thereon.

The Remedies, in general, are such as are easily procured, safely applied, and happily successful; being the result of many years experience—and first production of the kind in NEW-ENGLAND.

Intended for the use of

PRIVATE GENTLEMEN AND FARMERS.

By PAUL JEWETT, OF ROWLEY.

NEW EDITION, WITH VALUABLE ADDITIONS.

EXETER:
PUBLISHED BY JOSIAH RICHARDSON.
1826.

INTRODUCTION.

The subsequent treatise owes its rise to three principal causes.

I. The great opportunity I had, whilst young, of reading authors on Farriery, and thereby gaining an extensive theory.

II. The extensive practice I have had in this kind of business since, and the reasons experience hath given me, to differ from most of the European theories, and confine my practice to observation only.

III. The solicitations of my acquaintance.

In a work of this kind, I cannot be so particular in my prescriptions for cures as I am in my daily practice: The constitutions of beasts being different, will require some difference in the treatment, which must be directed by the judgment of those who are present.

I shall, in the first place, make some remarks on the choice of seed horses, and treatment of horses in general. On the management of colts till three years old, and at first riding them. Directions for docking, nicking, &c.—Likewise, of the various maladies with which they are affected.

Secondly, I shall treat of the various diseases affecting Neat Cattle. Sheep and Swine, in the next place, will claim our attention.

PART I.

OF SEED HORSES, AND THE MANAGEMENT OF COLTS.

Such seed horses should be chosen as are large and well proportioned, strait limbed, moving in a right line, heedless of every thwarting object, of an even persevering temper, with short fine hair and lively countenance.

Colts, when they are foaled, require but little attention the first three or four months. When they are weaned (if by grass) they should be kept in a small inclosure, with a constant supply of water, and tender herbage: If they are weaned by hay, provide yourself with a quantity of rowin or second crop hay; which is a grateful fodder for their tender years, and easily masticated; while coarse hay would be neglected, and your colt starved.

Colts of the first and second year, are frequently troubled with the lampers, being a fleshy excresence, or spongy substance, growing in the roof of the mouth, and hindering the colt from chewing. The best method of curing this inconvenience is, by applying a hot iron with a round head, till it is burnt so as to flow off; and in a few days it is well.

Give your colt a good pasture till he is three or four years old, then you must apply your rules of instruction to form the horse's manners; for (as the wise man says, in another case) train him up in the way he should go, and he will not forget it all his days.

A horse is a tractable animal, and is subjected to many servile employments, when used with gentleness and good humour; yet they remember injuries, and have recollection to avoid appearances which once gave them pain. A horse that stumbles (and 'tis a good horse that never stumbles) if he is frequently chastised for it, will at the least mistep, exert himself to an uncommon degree, fearing the lash, and often plunges himself and rider to the earth. This conduct must arise from the remembrance of his stripes, on similar occasions.

If your horse espies an object of fear in his way, heighten not the sensation with a whip or harsh words; for he will presently imagine them all connected, and double his flight. Gentlemen who intend a horse for the carriage, should familiarise him to the harness in some coach or wagon, where he cannot get away, till he submits himself tamely to be checked and forwarded at pleasure.

I now think it proper to give a few directions relative to docking, nicking, &c.

The curtailing of horses is both ornamental and useful; a long tail, if the roads are muddy, gathers much dirt, and impedes the horse's travelling. Many horses of worth make but little figure on account of their low carriage; the elevation of the tail therefore, is the object of enquiry. For this purpose the horse should be cast on some easy spot, that you may act with caution, then place a block under the tail, and hold your dividing instrument obliquely, so as to cut the under sinews the shortest; then their antagonists acting with superior force, will elevate the tail. Should the arteries bleed profusely, sear them with a hot iron, and anoint the sore every day with some emolient ointment, till it is well.

If nicking is thought necessary, the horse must be cast as for docking; the apparatus being ready, which should be a phlegm knife, a small pair of pincers, an iron spatula, and a cup of warm spirits: then with your knife, make an incision upon the cord of the tail which lies on each side of the bone, one inch and a half long, four inches from the body; the cord appearing, take hold of it with your pincers and run the spatula under it, then cut the cord at the upper part of the incision next the body, and do the same by the other cord. Then at two inches from your former incision, towards the end of the tail, cut down upon the cords as before, and take away four inches of each cord, or if it is thought necessary, the whole of the cord may be taken away in the same manner. Now apply your spirit, and bind up the sore with a linen bandage; unbind the horse and put him into a very narrow stable, fix a pulley over his back, put a line through and tie one end to the horse's tail, with a sufficient weight on the other end, to keep the tail upright; wet it daily with spirit, and apply some digestive, such as basilicon, and in ten or fifteen days you may expect a cure.

OBSERVATIONS ON PRESERVING HEALTH.

HEALTH, is that state of the animal body, in which all the functions relative thereto, are performed with ease and agility; the food received, is duly assimilated to the nourishment of the body, the fluids have a free, and equable round of circulation, and the fibres or nervous system, which is accounted the spring of sensation and motion, are not become rigid and inelastic; which would give rise to every species of inflammatory affection; neither flaxed, lax or weak, which would indulge a decline, and soon put a period to his existence.

In order therefore, to secure a horse in a state of health, and prevent a train of ills, we must have a special regard to him, with respect to food, exercise and stabling.

The intent of this treatise is, not to lose sight of the main object, while we are busying with unnecessary details—those who are fond of prolixity may consult Clark's Farrier on the subject.

I shall now lay before my readers, the several sorts of fodder and grain, used for horses, with the choice of each.

The principal hay for horses is herds grass and clover: the grain, oats, rye, barley, corn, bran, potatoes, &c. Some farmers, indeed, can support their horses on meadow or salt hay; but I presume, unless grain is substituted for better fodder, such horses are unfit for daily and laborious exercise; and if required, ten to one, he quits the servile scene, and leaves May verdant hills for happier brutes.

Herds grass, if well made, is the best fodder; it is more nutritious according to its weight than clover. Horses however are extremely fond of clover, and it keeps the bowels loose, but if indulged their fill, and immediately put to exercise, it may be of bad consequence, and often bring on what is called the phthisic. Farmers frequently feed their horses through the winter on corn fodder; it is very good if rightly managed.

A horse is an animal of a hot constitution, and

especially when fed on dry meat, is subject to costiveness—this should be guarded against by gentle laxatives—A mess of potatoes every day, or a mash of bran, or boiled rye, will generally keep the bowels loose, and secure your horse from those complaints, which counterfeit the bots, or another disorder which is called the dry belly-ache. Oats, the common provender for horses in our country, contain a latent spirit which supports the beast under great fatigue, and encourages them to the most sevile employment with the greatest freedom; yet if a small portion of corn should be added to every feed of oats, they would probably be broken much finer, and consequently be more nutritious. Barley is also very grateful to horses, but much the best ground. In feeding your horses, whether you serve up the hay in a manger or rack, be careful to give no more than your horse will eat with a good appetite; lest suffering to breathe upon, and spoil the sweetness of his hay, you imagine him sick, and either send him to the Farrier, or take some method with him, that will make him truly sick. Give your horse therefore often, and but little at a time; let his water also be given him when he craves; some horses are more thirsty than others, and unless indulged with water, will refuse the choicest hay. There is likewise a great choice in water. Those waters that readily mix with alkaline substances and common soap, are best suited to dilute the food, and promote the secretions of an animal body.

ON EXERCISE.

A HORSE that hath been used to labour, or suffered to roam abroad, is an unsuitable subject for confinement, especially if his manner of living becomes more luxurious. Idleness brings on a redundency of the fluids, and a congestion of that perspirable matter, thrown off by exercise.

When this therefore is detained in the body, it will prove a stimulus to many general and local diseases. I have seen it verified in many instances of gentlemen's horses, who afford them leisure, and are not careful to apply that excellent substitute friction, or currying.

I now find a necessity of changing my advice, and advocating the wretchedness of those animals, whose silent groans demand our commisseration.

Horses cannot travel through heat and rain, over the sandy heath or rocky mountain, insensible as the chariot to which he is harnessed. The rider should make his stages, as the difficulty of the way and strength of the animal indicates. His limbs should be rubbed with a brush or woollen cloth, to prevent their growing stiff and swelling; he should not be permitted to drink till cool, and in dusty weather his hay should be sprinkled with water, and his grain soaked at all seasons of the year. But these remarks will more properly occur, when I shall give directions for travelling horses.

All I need say further in this place is, consider what your beast is capable of performing, and the keeping you bestow on him; then require no more than reason exacts, and you may expect a long and faithful servant.

A REMARK OR TWO ON STABLES.

THE stabling of horses in the country, requires but few directions, their stables in general being capacious enough for a free circulation of air, which is as necessary for a horse, as for the human species. But where thirty or forty are kept together in a close stable, where the air has no access but by the door, together with the sharp exhalations from the urine, perspiration of their bodies, &c. it renders the situation disagreeable, and almost intolerable. A horse in health, to remain long in such a place, would soon be enervated and unfit for business. Stables should be situated where the air may have a draught through them; and in every horse's apartment a small window should be placed, and left open through the night, and not shut up to suffocate its inhabitants, as too frequently is the case in sea-port towns.

I shall now discourse upon the principal general disorders, to which horses are incident; next of local diseases, which will be connected with those of surgery.

GLANDERS OR HORSE AIL.

This disease is justly called the glanders, being principally an affection of the glands of the head; but from its frequent appearance, it is vulgarly called the horse ail.

You will perceive this disease by the sadness of the horse's countenance, loss of appetite, difficulty in drinking, and sudden debility of strength. Frequently the glands under the jaws are swelled and in an advanced stage of the disease, there will be a continual discharge of thin ichorous matter from the nose.

The remedies are these. Let blood freely in the mouth, or by perforating the nose with a sharp awl; put him under a course of physic, by giving him brimstone, antimony and turmerick in succession for two weeks. Let a dose be given him every day in a mess of bran. The dose of brimstone and turmerick, half an ounce each; that of antimony, one fourth of an ounce. Put a rowel in his breast, and then strive to bring the swelling under his throat, to a suppuration, by applying emolient poultices and fomenting baths. When the swelling becomes soft, and the matter fluctuating, place a ceton in the most depending part, to discharge the humour. Fumigate his head twice a day, with sulphur and camphire mixed with rye paste, dried, and burnt under his nose; likewise scraps of old leather— and occasionally blow snuff up his nose. If the discharge of matter becomes thick, white and mild, you may soon expect a cure.

FRENZY OR STAGGERS.

This disease is known by a hanging down of the head, watery eyes, and reeling of the body. From the general cause of this disease we infer the method of cure. The excretions are diminished, consequently a costiveness and induration of the contents of the intestines, seems the cause. The horse must be bled the first day in the neck, the third day in the mouth; give him the first day, four quarts of herb drink, made of mallows and flax seed, to lubricate his bowels, and prepare for a dose of aloes; one ounce and a half of which is to be given him the second day to purge him. The third day bleed in the mouth as before; the fourth, give him the following nourishing decoction: Take two quarts of ale, boil in it a white loaf crust, or hard biscuit; when taken from the fire, add one gill of honey, and give it to the horse luke-warm; put a plaster of pitch upon his temples: Be sure to keep him in a dark stable, and let his food be given him sparingly.

YELLOWS.

This disease in horses is similar to the jaundice in men. It arises from obstructions formed in the biliaryducts, which prevents the bile from flowing into the stomach, but forces it to return into the circulation, which gives that yellow appearance in the white of the eyes and urine, and that sense of weariness to the limbs in the animal diseased.

Cure.—Take aloes, venetian soap and honey equal quantities, to be made into pills, and half an ounce given daily for a week. If this does not effect a cure, steep celandine and saffron in cider, to be given one quart a day. It is often necessary in this disease to let blood.

STRANGURY OR DIFFICULTY OF STALEING.

Many causes may produce this disease, such as over fatigue or catching cold; which brings on a stricture in the renal vessels, and consequently an obstruction of urine. Another frequent cause is, driving the beast too long without suffering him to stop and stale.

Cure.—Take one ounce of nitre and dissolve it in one quart of ale or beer, to be given the horse blood warm; or a pint of juniper berries boiled in two quarts of fair water to the consumption of one half, and given warm; half an ounce of rosin pounded and given in meal a few days will perform wonders.

FEVER.

To judge of the state of the fever, you may examine the pulse; which your will find in thin skined horses, by pressing your fingers gently on the temporal artery, about an inch and a quarter backward from the upper corner of the eye; or in the inside of the leg, just above the knee. But you may be better satisfied, by putting your hands to the horse's nostrils, and judging from the heat of his breath.

CURE.—In the beginning of a fever, it is generally necessary to let blood, but in an advanced state, when the heat is great, and the discharge from the bowels diminished, or the dung hard and dry, glysters are also necessary.

For a glister or clyster.

Take one handful of mallows, boil in milk and water, also two spoonfuls of flax-seed; and add to it, when boiled, half a pound of sugar, and as much sweet oil, with a handful of salt; then with the necessary apparatus, put it up the horse's body.

You must also observe, a cooling regimen. Take a four pail pot and hang over your fire, full of water, and clover or honey-suckle hay; make a tea of it. When your horse is thirsty, let him drink it luke warm. Then take a quart of this liquor and dissolve in it one ounce of nitre, to be given morning and evening, till the fever abates. Let his hay, if he will eat, be sprinkled with warm water, and his provender soaked.

CRAMP OR DRAWING OF THE NERVES.

THIS is a disease I have never read of, but have had many instances of it in my practice. The almost only cause, is taking cold after hard labour and sweating. The excresions being suddenly diminished, brings on these spasmodic and convulsive symptoms. Upon the least motion, every nerve seems contracted, to overthrow its

B

antagonist, and as it were to dismember its ungovernable body. The eyes are contorted in their sockets, and they are blind except by accident, and nothing but the white appears.

The method I have found of uncommon efficacy, is this. Immediately take a pound and half of blood from the jugular; then place your horse in a warm stable, and prepare to sweat him. Take a large pot, and fill it with May-weed and tansy; when boiled place it under the horse's belly, and cover him with a large coverlet, to keep the steam of the bath confined to the body. A little previous to the bath, give him fifteen or eighteen grains of opium in half a pint of wine. Now take special care that the cold be not repeated; let him wear his covering a day or two, and carry him his water moderately warm. This method has proved salutary many times, and seems to have its reason in the nature of things.

HAVING attended briefly to the more general distempers, I shall call my readers' attention to the more partial or local inconveniences, to which horses are subject. As I purpose brevity, I shall not enter into theoretical, or physical disputations on the subject, but strive to discover simple truth in a simple manner.

FISTULA.

THE fistula is an ulcer of the callous kind, and from its well known fatality to horses, is generally supposed incurable. I confess there are few diseases more stubborn, yet must remark, that neglect of means, or wrong applications have in ten instances to one, been the cause of my ill success. Its seat in horses is between the sadder and collar; which are commonly the source from which it arises. Bruises of any kind may produce it. From its position on the top of the withers, the matter when collected, instead of being discharged, corrodes and insinuates between the cords of the neck, from which it can hardly be eradicated. Most people apply clay mixed with vinegar, to the surface of the sore, to dry it up; which might answer well, where a good drain is opened; but here it proves a source of deception, and while you anticipate a cure, your horse is ruined.

My method of cure is this; first with a limber probe, search the bottom of the sore, see whether it is sinuous or hollow; find the direction of the sinews, whether it runs between the shoulder blades, or only on one side. When you have made sufficient search into the depth of the sore, and find it curable, you must prepare to make a drain from the bottom : and this must be done either by the knife or rowel.

Observation.—Where the rowel will answer, never take the knife; for, by destroying the teguments, you make a large sore, cause great pain to the beast, and protract the cure. If roweling, therefore, is proposed, make one of hair, put it through the eye of a crooked needle; put your needle to the bottom of the sore, and thrust it through in a depending manner, that the discharge may be easy; stir it frequently, and wash the sore with strong lye, or soap-suds, to keep it clean.— If fungous flesh arises, sprinkle it with blue stone, or red precipitate; and sometimes fill the sore with lime or ashes, which will help the digestion, and cleanse the sore. If the sore is filled with a callous pipe, and appears of long standing; the knife or hot iron must be applied.

The horse being cast on an easy spot, with a

knife or hot iron, as most convenient, you must take away the callous or fungous flesh; if it should bleed profusely, melt some rosin on the sore with a hot-iron, and sear the arteries. Lay a cloth upon the sore wet with spirit, and unbind your horse; if an inflammation succeeds, supple it with a hot bath, to reduce the swelling, and bring on a suppuration. Now, be careful to keep it from the air, and apply your digestive, made of basilicon; and if proud or fungous flesh is seen, add to it a little verdigrise. Yet, if after all your care, the matter falls between the shoulder-blades, or upon the neck bone, so that no drain can be made from the bottom of the sore; you had better give up the cure, and save your trouble.

Horses often have swellings upon their shoulders, that are not sinuous; in such cases, bathing with hot vinegar or urine will generally make a resolution of the humour, and prevent further mischief.

SHOULDER STRAIN.

This lameness is brought on by overstraining the limb. There is a collection of grumous blood between the shoulder-blade and body; the small vessels being over-extended or ruptured by the strain, is the cause of the extravasated fluid, which must be re-absorbed or drained off, before the beast will get well.

Cure.—My method of cure is this: Take up a piece of skin on the corner of the shoulder, as large as a nine pence, then put your finger to the hole, and start the skin from the flesh two inches round, and blow up the shoulder. Now put in a piece of leather, cut round, with a hole in the middle, answering to that in the shoulder. This in about twelve or fifteen days, will discharge the humour, and being taken out, will seldom fail of a cure.

This method has been reprobated by some; but experience has taught me to adopt it. Where the lameness is slight, I have found the following an efficacious remedy:

Take of high wines one pint, oil of spike one gill, pigs' feet oil one gill, gum camphor half an ounce, and one beasts gall. Simmer these together over a gentle fire, apply it warm to the diseased part, and heat it in with a dish of coals or hot slice, twice in a day.

CLAP IN THE BACK SINEWS.

This disease is a lameness in the back sinews, between the knee and fetlock joint. It is produced by a strain, which debilitates the nerves, and therefore produces lameness. The cords of the leg will sometimes swell, which will determine the seat of the disease; if not, you may know it from a shoulder strain by the horse's steping short, but taking his foot from the ground; whereas, in a shoulder strain, the horse will drag his toe on the ground when he walks.

Cure.—This may be easily effected, by bathing the leg in the day time, with the ointment prescribed for a shoulder strain; at night apply an emollient poultice of turnips and Indian meal. Make a boot for the horse's leg, tie it at the fetlock, then fill it with your poultice, and tie it again above the knee. This method followed a few days, will prove an efficacious remedy.

HIDE BOUND.

This is brought on by low keeping and surfeits; the juices of the body are dissipated, the skin becomes rigid, and as it were adheres to the ribs.——To cure this inconvenience, it will be necessary to put your horse on a more liberal diet; also every day a mash of bran or boiled rye should be given him; and twice a week give him half an ounce of brimstone in his bran.

BROKEN WIND.

HORSES by over riding, especially when their bellies are full of water, or clover hay, have their wind hurt, and are called broken winded. The cure is difficult. Take of tar and honey one spoonful each; liquorish ball, half the quantity; opium, eight grains; mix and dissolve them in a quart of new milk, to be given every morning fasting. Let his water be that wherein quick lime has been slacked; the proportion is a pint of lime to a pail of water.

Feed him as much as possible on arse-smart hay, which has been sprinkled with warm water.

BOTTS AND WORMS.

THE signs that indicate the botts, are uneasy motions in the horse, frequently turning his head to his sides, often lying down, or scouring of the guts.

CURE.—Sweeten one quart of milk with honey, and give it to the horse with a horn; then powder half an ounce of aloes, and give it directly in a strong decoction of savine bows; if they have not eaten through the intestines, you may depend on a cure. Tobacco leaves cut fine, or coarse horse hair, and mixed with a horse's provender, will prevent botts and worms from collecting in the maw; and will often kill them.

GRIPES.

THIS disease hath similar symptons with the botts; it arises from sudden colds, indurated dung and spasms of the intestines. If you are not sure whether botts are the cause, take this method first, which will often destroy them:

Give the horse three gills of gin, with as much sweet oil; if he is costive, give him an ounce of aloes, made into balls with castile soap and honey. If this does not work, give him a glister made of tobacco leaves steeped in old urine, and sweetened with molasses; these remedies are adapted as near as possible, to suit both disorders.

SCOURING.

This is brought on by drinking too much cold water, or by eating sour hay, &c.

Cure.—Give your horse two quarts of the liquor, wherein garden rhubarb, flax seed and mallows, have been boiled; or boil white oak bark, and white pine together; give him one quart of this morning and evening till well.

SORE BACK.

If the skin is wore off a horse's back, and the sides of the sore are swelled, bathe it with hot urine, or with salt and water; this will disperse the swelling. If you wish to dry up the sore, powder chalk, or old shoes burnt, and cover the sore with it. If his back is full of hard lumps, or what is commonly called saddle boils, bleed him freely in the mouth, which will serve as a dose of physic; then wash his back often with hot rum and vinegar.

BLEEDING.

This is a resource which unskilful men fly to on every failure of their horse, without considering the nature of the disease, or state of the horse's body.

Proper subjects for bleeding.

Horses that are affected with any inflammatory disorder, whether general or topical, as fevers, inflamed sores, or any hot humour, are proper subjects for bleeding. Horses that are fat and plethoric, require more frequent bleeding than those of the opposite state; but observe not to deprive them of the vital fluid beyond necessity; rather bleed often, and but little at a time. Horses that are poor have no fluid to spare, rather recruit them by a generous diet and leisure.

Unskilful grooms, when they bleed in the jugular, often cut through the vein; whence an extravasation of the blood, and no small danger to the horse.

Among many other instances, the Honourable *Benjamin Greenleaf, Esq.* sent me a horse in this condition. I ordered his servant to apply the simple remedy of cold water, liberally, and in a few days he was cured.

PRICKED OR GRAVELED HOOFS.

Horses are sometimes pricked in shoeing, it will fester, and cause the horse to be lame; extract the nail and fill up the hole with the horse-ointment, to be mentioned by and by. Sometimes gravel will get into the nail hole, or into cracks in the hoofs; unless this is soon extracted it will remain long in the hoof, and spoil the horse's usefulness. Many by cutting the hoof to get out the gravel, make the remedy worse than the disease; if you cannot find the gravel with a little cutting, make a poultice of turnips and put the horse's foot into it; repeat this a few days and the gravel will generally work out.

Note—if you omit this practice too long, the horse will not be cured till the gravel works out the top of the hoof.

The Horse Ointment.

Take yellow rosin, bees-wax and honey, like quantities; hog's lard and turpentine, double their quantity; melt them all together over a gentle fire, and keep a continual stiring: when they are well compounded, take it from the fire and stir in a little verdigrese.

This is an excellent ointment for sores, burns, bruises, choped heels, &c.

SPAVINS.

THERE are three sorts of spavins. First, the bone spavin; it is a bony excrescence formed on the joint, which impedes the motion of the joint, and is seldom curable.

Secondly, the wind spavin; it commonly comes in the horse's ham. Prick the swelling with a phlegm knife, but take special care not to injure the nervous cords, for this will often bring on the lock-jaw. Upon opening the swelling, you will often find a gelatinous humour to issue from the opening; now apply your turnip poultice for a few days to suck out the humour; then strengthen the part, by bathing it with good brandy.

Thirdly, the blood spavin. The coats of the vein being ruptured, the blood extravasates and forms a protuberance in the vein.

CURE.—Take up the vein with a crooked needle, and tie it above the swelling; then let blood below it, and apply cow-dung fryed in goose grease and vinegar, by way of poultice.

SPLENT.

SPLENTS are of the same nature with spavins, but not upon the joints. They are bony excrescences of an oblong figure, coming between the fettock joint and knee, or gambrel; while they are growing, they make the horse lame, but when they are formed, unless they press upon the cords of the leg, they are of very little damage.

Cure.—Shave the part and put on a smart blistering plaister, to be kept on three days; chafe the part strongly with the tincture of flies; and once a day rub in oppodeldoc with one quarter part oil of turpentine; this will generally effect a cure, if curable.

WIND-GALLS.

These appear upon the fettocks, and are the consequence of hard riding. They are full of wind or jelly, they seldom lame a horse, and may be cured in the same manner that wind spavins are.

RING-BONE.

This is a long callous just above the hoof, if long neglected, the hoof will become narrow and twist, and often prove incurable.

I have cured many recent ring-bones in the following manner:—Make a boot for the horse's foot, tie it at the top of the hoof, then take oyster shell lime, newly burned, and fill the boot against the ring-bone with the lime; place the horse's foot in a tub of water, or in a pond of standing water; repeat this five days; after this, poultice the foot for five days more with a turnip poultice and linseed oil; observing to chafe the part before you apply the poultice. Lastly, apply a plaister of pitch to the ring-bone, to be worn two or three weeks. This method hath succeeded with the greater half I have tried. Those who use stone lime, may expect a fire that he cannot extinguish, for by this, many have ruined their horses.

SORE EYES.

If the eyes are much inflamed, let blood in the neck, then boil the bark of bass wood root with rose leaves, sweeten the decoction with loaf sugar, wash the horse's eyes three times a day with this water, and keep him in a dark stable. If films grow over the eye, dissolve ten grains of white vitirol, and as much rock allum, in a gill of spring water; dip a feather into it, and touch the eye a few days with it, and it will eat away the film.

SCRATCHES.

Horses are troubled with these most frequently in the spring, while the roads are muddy, which obstructs the perspiration of the parts; together with the snow water, which is very unfavourable to this disorder.

Cure.—Cut the hair off close, and wash the legs with strong soap suds or urine; put on a turnip poultice (as this is the best I know of for horses) a few days, mixed with hog's fat and linseed oil; it will soon effect a cure.

FILING TEETH.

When horses are old, their fore teeth grow long, while their jaw teeth wear short; this prevents the horses from grinding their hay; and by that means they grow poor and die, before their natural vigour is exhausted. To remedy this inconvenience, and prolong a serviceable life, provide a gag to put in his mouth, then a coarse file—having gaged your horse, file his fore teeth so short that his grinders may touch, and break the hardest hay.

This is an easy and certain method of making old horses eat their hay equal to young ones; provided their jaw teeth are sound.

STIFLE.

The stifle joint is above the inside bend of the hough or gambrel; its use is much the same as the knee-pan in man. If the stifle is only strained, bathe it with the ointment prescribed for strains in the hip; which will soon cure it. If it is dislocated, or out of place, make a stifle shoe, in form of a cone—let a natural shoe be the base; then, with three pieces of iron, one from the toe, the other two from the sides of the shoe, to meet in a point three inches from the base. Put this upon the well foot, that the horse may stand upon the lame one four or five days; that will keep the joint in place—and in the mean time bathe the part with the ointment above mentioned. Note—The stifle shoe is preferable to straping the well leg, for straping hinders the circulation, brings off the hair, and often lames the well leg.

STRAINS IN THE HIP.

Horses are frequently lame in the hip; this is occasioned by the ligament which holds the thigh bone into the socket, being overstretched. To effect a cure, the horse must have but little exercise, and the joint should be bathed three times a day, with three parts of brandy, and one of oil of spike, to be heat in by a chafing-dish of coals; this will contract and strengthen the ligament, and if a recent lameness, will prove a certain remedy.

HIPED AND HALF HIPED.

When the bones of the hip fall so low as to be called hiped, the horse becomes useless; but when they are only half-hiped, or hip-shot, the hip may be strengthened, and the horse (though disfigured) may perform much labour.

CURE.—Take white oak bark, elm and white pine bark; roots, Solomon-seal, buck horn and comfrey; boil them all together, and frequently bathe the hip with it; this in a little time will strengthen the hip and fit the horse for business.

HOOF BOUND.

Hoofs that are hard, dry, and withal contracted at the top so as to pinch upon the quick, and prevent a free circulation, are said to be hoof bound. To prevent this, keep the hoofs cool and moist; to cure it, take a phlegm lancet, and open the hoof at the edge of the hair, to give it liberty of spreading. Then grease it daily with woodchuck, skunk or dog's grease, that it may grow.

A few Directions for Choosing a Horse.

THERE is much pleasure and profit in the service of a good horse, but very little of either in a bad one. There are many mean horses that make a good appearance when taken from the hand of a jockey. In purchasing a horse, then, trust not too much to the seller's word; let your own judgment, or that of a friend, be chiefly relied on. See that he hath good feet and joints, and that he stands well on his legs; see that his fore teeth shut even, for many horses have their under jaw the shortest; these will grow poor at grass. See that his hair is short and fine, for this denotes a good horse. Observe his eyes, that they are clear and free from blemishes, that they are not moon eyed, or white eyed, for such are apt to start in the night. A large hazel coloured eye is the best.

Look at his knees, see that the hair or skin is not broken, for this denotes a stumbler. Take care that his wind is good; for a trial of this, let him be fed on good hay for twenty-four hours, take him then to water, and let him drink his fill; place him with his head the lowest, if then he will breathe free, there is no danger. See that his countenance is bright and cheerful; this is an excellent mirror to discover his goodness in. If his nostrils are broad, it is a sign that he is well winded; narrow nostrils the contrary.

See that his spirits are good, but that he is gentle and easily governed; not inclined to start.— In travelling, mind that he lifts his feet neither too high or too low; that he does not interfere or overreach, and that he carries his hind legs the widest. See that he is well ribbed back, and not high boned. The size may be determined by the purchaser. Age, from five to ten is the best. There are many tricks practised by jockies, to make horses appear young, but it is not consistent with the size of my book, to detect them; all I would say is, that horses' teeth when young are wide, white and even; the inside of their mouths are fleshy, and their lips hard and firm. On the contrary, the mouth of an old horse is lean above and below, the lips are soft and easily turned up; their teeth grow longer, narrower, and of a yellow colour.

REMARKS ON TRAVELLING.

According to my promise, I shall give my readers a few directions relative to travelling horses. If you are to take a long journey, you must prepare your horse by good feeding and gentle exercise. A horse that is exhausted with hard labour, advanced in age, or very young, will not bear the fatigues of a long journey.— Neither will a very fat horse, or one who has lived without exercise, be a fit subject for travelling. A horse, therefore, rather meager than fat, used to active exercise, whose flesh is firm from good living and labour, is the most likely to answer your expectation. Some days before your journey, have him shod, lest being pricked with a nail, he fail you on the road. Look well to his saddle, and see it fits with ease, and does not hurt his back; and while upon the road examing it daily, and repair it as needed.

Before your horse eats in the morning, give him a little water, that he may eat the better; but do not lead him to the trough or brook till you take him out for riding; the water now taken into the stomach, will better dilute the food; and by washing his mouth, prevent any sudden thirst on the road. Ride moderately while your horse's belly is full, for he will mend his pace as this fullness goes off.

Before you make a stage, restrain your horse, and take him in cool; let him eat a little hay before he is watered, if hot; and thus conduct at all your stages. At night, after your horse is cooled, wash his legs with water, (warm water is best) for it promotes perspiration, cleanses away the sand, and prevents his legs from swelling. His back should likewise be washed, to prevent those little saddle boils which the friction of the saddle often produces. In the middle of the day, I should prefer a bating of hay to any grain; but let it be sprinkled, in warm weather, with water. New oats are not good for a horse on a journey; they make him faint, and often bring on a diarkea. If old oats cannot be had, (as is sometimes the case at harvest) feed him with Indian meal, or oat meal. Horses on a journey, from their increased perspiration, and constant feeding on dry meat, are apt to be costive; to prevent this, give them occasionally a marsh of bran, or boiled rye.

If your horse discovers an inclination to stale on the road, let him stop for that purpose; and if the discharge is difficult, give him an ounce of nitre for a few nights in his provender. A horse hath not the faculty of speech, but subjects himself to his master, to whom he complains under every indisposition. Will not then reason, interest, and pity, prompt us to adopt the most approved methods for their welfare?

PART II.

OF THE DISEASES OF CATTLE.

CATTLE are subject to many diseases, at all seasons of the year, but more especially in the spring; which I shall endeavour in a brief manner to give an account of.

FEVER.

WHEN a fever takes place, the beast looses his appetite, the nose becomes dry, and the horns cold, the eyes appear dull and the countenance fallen.

In the beginning of the disease, one quart of blood should be taken from the jugular; but if the fever is far advanced, and a trembling or twitching of the muscles has taken place, to bleed would be dangerous, and often fatal. Boil fever-bush and angelica, like quantities; give the beast one gallon at a time twice a day, also one gill of sweet oil per day. The above dose is for an ox or cow; for lesser cattle, it must be in proportion.

MURRAIN.

This disorder comes under the nether jaw, the chaps swell, and upon search you find it full of a watery humour. This disease commonly happens to cattle that are thin of flesh.

Cure.—In the first place put a rowel through the most depending part of the swelling, to be stired frequently, then give the beast the following singular, but efficacious remedy.

Take half a pint of hen's dung, and dissolve in one quart of old urine, and cause the beast to drink it. This, if applied seasonably, will never fail of a cure.

COUGH OR SHORTNESS OF BREATH.

Cure.—Give the beast to drink divers mornings together, one spoonful of tar, and as much honey, dissolved in a quart of new milk, with one head of garlick bruised, and put in with it.

WIND CHOLIC.

This is discovered by the beast being very uneasy, lying down and getting up often, and frequently swelling very much.

Cure.—Take a quart of warm water and half a pint of gin, sweetened well with molasses, then put in half a pint of pounded mustard seed, pour it down, and drive the beast about and it will move the wind.

EOR THE SCAB OR SCURF.

Take soft soap and tar and anoint the place, and it will soon cure it.

FOR PISSING OF BLOOD.

Take milk and bring it to a curd with runnet, mix it with ash leaves and nettle seeds choped fine, and made into balls, to be put down the beast's throat.

BLADDERS.

This disease happens under the tongue, being a number of small bladders, full of a watery humour: the beast breathes with difficulty and drools at the mouth.

Cure.—The saline watery humour must be let out with an incision knife, or the bladders may be broken with your fingers. Then give the beast water to drink wherein bay salt and bay leaves have been concocted.

TAINT OR GARGET.

This is a hot humour that mostly affects cows' bags, but sometimes their limbs, and other cattle also.

Cure.—If the humour affects the cow's bag, the first thing to be done, is to take two pounds of blood from the neck, then put a piece of garget root in the double skin between the fore legs, with a hair rowel below that; when the humour subsides take the garget and rowel out, wash the bag three or four times a day with cold brine. If the swelling increases, scarify the skin and wash it with the brine of salt and urine.

If the garget affects the limbs, after bleeding, you must make a tea of horse-radish root, mustard seed and sage; give the beast two quarts at a time, daily, till well.

BLAINS.

This is a stoppage of the body, attended with a fever. It hath all the symptons of fever, such as dry nose, cold horns, &c. The body swells, and they make constant efforts to dung, but discharge little.

Cure.—Take away one quart of blood; then let some person skilled in the business, put his hand into the creature's body, after it is well greased, and take away the indurated dung; then such things as are physical must be given. First take one quart of chamber-lye, half a pint of molasses, with as much hog's lard, let them be simered together, then add a spoonful of gun-powder pounded, let it be put down the creature's throat with a horn. If the fever is not high, Hiera Picra is a good medicine, and the herb thoroughwort made into a strong tea, will often effect a cure.

FOR ANY POISONOUS THING EATEN.

Take milk, sallad oil and London treacle, mix them together and give it warm.

TO KILL WORMS.

Take savine, cut it fine and make it into balls, with fresh butter, to be put down the creature's throat. Or give half an ounce of powdered aloes in a quart of savine tea.

HORN AIL.

This disease is seated in the horns of cattle, the inside becomes carious, putrifies and is discharged from the nose. The beast that is taken with this disorder will frequently shake his head, and appear to be dizzy. If you would be sure of this disease, take a nail gimblet and perforate the horn, if it is hollow and no blood follows, it is the horn ail.

Cure.—Bore each horn into the hollow part, then inject into it strong vinegar and camphorated spiaits; this will cleanse the horn, and generally effect the cure.

OVERFLOWING OF THE GALL.

This distemper is similar to the jaundice in men, or the yellows in horses. The beasts grow suddenly weak, eat but little, often have a cough, their eyes and urine turn yellow.

Cure.—Any thing bitter is good, cherry tree bark, barberry bark, or celandine, steeped in cider, will generally effect a cure.

CATTLES' TEETH THAT ARE LOOSE.

Cure.—Rub their teeth well with fine salt, and it will fasten them.

BARBS IN THE MOUTH.

These are little white protuberances growing on the inside of the cheeks. In their natural state they are about one third of an inch long, but when they grow to such a length as to get between the teeth and turn blue, the beast will not eat, but grows poor and slavers at the mouth.

Cure.—Cut the barbs with a pair of scissors, and rub them with fine salt, which will soon cure them.

TO STOP VOMITING.

Boil tansy and mint together; give one quart of this to the beast. If it does not stop in an hour, give the same quantity again, and repeat it till stopped.

FOR LOSS OF THE CUD.

When cattle loose the cud, they will not masticate their food the second time, as they usually do; neither will they eat with an appetite.

Cure.—The quickest and best method is to take half the cud from another creature, and put it warm into the mouth of that which hath lost it; this remedy is infallible.

TO CURE WENS.

Wens, except those that are stifasts, are easily cured. When they appear to be ripe, put a hair rowel through the middle of them, and put on daily soft soap.

BROKEN HORNS.

Cattle, by many accidents, may have their horns broken, and unless proper methods are taken with them, they either loose their horns, or have them grow in a very unnatural manner.

Cure.—If they are not broken so as to come off from the frith, or even if they are, I have often cured them, by replacing them quickly, and making use of the following method.—Take a piece of wood and put across the horns to keep them their usual width; then put another piece in the middle of the former, to rest upon the forehead, bringing the horns in their natural position: lastly, prepare a bandage two or three yards long, four inches wide, to be dipped in strong pitch, while warm; when this is cold, it will keep the horn very firm, and being left on for three or four weeks, it will get perfectly well.

BROKEN LEGS.

The farther a leg is broken from the joint the better: fractures in the hip are seldom cured.

CURE.—Take Solomon seal root, buck horn and comfrey roots, each a handful, to be boiled in tar for a kniting plaister to be placed next the leg; then splinter it in the proper place, and with your narrow bandage bind it up, let it remain till it is well. It is sometimes necessary to sling the beast, that he may not misplace the leg by standing.

TAPING.

When cattle are swelled very much, it is often necessary to reduce them by taping. Take a sharp knife, gage it about an inch, and pierce the belly of the beast just below the short ribs, (always on the left side) then either keep the knife in and press it sideways, or put in a quill that the wind may extricate itself.

FALLING DOWN OF THE MATRICE OR REED.

Cows just before or after calving, if they are weak and suffered to lie with their hinder parts the lowest, sometimes have their reed protrubed or inverted. When this has happened and the part is swelled or torn, (for hens will pick and tear it to pieces, if they are suffered to) wash it with warm milk and water, to cleanse it of the filth and dirt; then boil a strong decoction of white oak or some other astringent bark, and bathe the part till it is contracted so as to be replaced in the body. Give the cow half a pint of brandy with a nutmeg grated in it as a cordial; prepare her bedding so that her hinder parts may lay the highest, and ring her up with three strong wire rings.

Sewing them up with a good waxed end, taking a deep stitch, will be much better than ringing or bandages.

CALVING.

Cows sometimes need assistance to bring forth their young; if they have strength, the situation of the calf may make it difficult, if not impracticable. Naturally, a calf presents its fore feet and head first; but if this is not the case, and the head of the calf is fallen below the bones, the hand must be introduced into the body, and push the calf back, and withal raise his head above the bones, then he may be taken away with ease. If the calf should be inverted and present his tail first, the hand should be put into the cow's body and the calf turned if possible. If that cannot be done, you may endeavour to bring it away by the hind legs, which may be done many times with ease. The cow should stand, if she hath strength, which will greatly facilitate the delivery. The secundine, or cleansing, should be taken away directly after the calf, for if suffered to remain long in the body, it is attended with many bad consequences.

PERFORATING COWS DUGS.

It sometimes happens that cows when they calve, have their dugs knotted, and the passage through them becomes impervious, they consequently give no milk. To remedy this inconvenience, make a small skewer of walnut or whalebone, and force it up the middle of the dug; take it out daily and anoint it with goose grease, do thus till it heals round the skewer. I have been successful in many attempts of this kind, and would recommend it as the best method in cases of this sort.

CALVES THAT SCOUR.

Young calves are subject to a looseness or scouring.

CURE.—Take a pint of new milk, and put two spoonfuls of rennet into it, to be put immediately down the calves stomach, this forming a curd in the stomach will prevent the flux.

CATTLE THAT ARE OVERHEAT.

I HAVE frequently seen cattle, especially oxen, that from two much fatigue in hot weather, were what some call melted, or overheat. This brings on such a relaxed state of the solids that nature will seldom restore them to their primitive tone. The circulation being impeded (which always succeeds overheating) consequently the perspiration is diminished and retained, and the beast remains an inactive drone for life.

CURE.—Give the beast directly one quart of gin, or for want of that W. India rum; this acting as a stimulus, will strengthen the solids, quicken the fluids, promote all the secretions, and very generally effect a cure.

TAIL SICK.

CATTLE in the spring season, more especially young ones, are what is commonly called tail sick. The end of the tail for some inches becomes loose and spongy, the creature looses its appetite, and is sick. The simple remedy is, cut off the tail above the loose part, and it will form a cure.

BLEEDING.

THE best time to bleed is in the spring of the year and increase of the moon. Old cattle require oftener bleeding than young ones; but the quantity should be less. Cattle you intend to fat, should be bled three or four months successively, in the first part of the year, in the increase of the moon, and but little at a time. In all other cases you must bleed as the exigences of the case require, and as mentioned in the various diseases.

PART III.

OF SHEEP.

A SHEEP, perhaps, is one of the most useful animals of our country: their annual fleece being manufactured at home, or in our now flourishing woollen manufactories, afford us a neat and comfortable apparel; their flesh a wholesome food for our tables.

Sheep are of a hot nature, and require to be kept cool; they should not be housed, except in rainy weather. Ewes, before they lamb, should have corn, beans or turnips every day, which will enable them to bring forth their young with vigour. After they have lambed, a few potatoes every day will make a flow of milk: if they should bring on a looseness, give them corn instead of potatoes.

Sheep should be sheared, the moon increasing; their wool will be longer and better: some shear their lambs in August, affirming that the succeeding fleece is not the less for it. Sheep should be washed in the spring with a decoction of tobacco; this will kill the ticks, and prevent their rubbing the wool off.

I shall now enumerate some of the maladies to which sheep are subject.

PLAGUE.

Wash the sheep in alum and salt water, and give them to drink a decoction of rue and balm leaves.

TO CURE POISON.

WHEN snow falls before you have taken up your sheep, they often, through force of hunger, eat winter-green, which will make them froth at the mouth and swell, and in a little time die.

Cure.—Take a gill of sweet oil, or for want of that, hog's fat or fresh butter; mix it with a pint of new milk to be given to the sheep; if it is taken seasonably it will effect a cure.

LOSS OF THE CUD.

TAKE the cud from another sheep and divide it between the two, or mix clay in urine with the powder of alum, make it up in little balls and put one or two down the sheep's throat, and after it a half a pint of vinegar.

TO INCREASE MILK.

IN the spring give the ewes beans, corn, or potatoes, and in the summer change of pasture; this will increase the milk, and make the lambs grow well.

FOR THE SCAB OR ITCH.

ANOINT the part affected with tar and fresh butter, mixed together, or wash the sheep in pennyroyal water, and it will preserve them from the scab.

FEVER IN SHEEP.

DISSOLVE half an ounce of nitre in water and vinegar, and give it to the sheep luke-warm.

TO KILL MAGGOTS IN SHEEP.

MIX tar and goose grease, equal quantities, and stir in flower of sulphur, as much as to make it of a proper consistence, anoint the place with the ointment, and it will kill them.

FOR A COUGH.

TAKE colts foot, lung wort, and maiden hair, boil them to a strong tea, sweeten it with honey, and give it the sheep to drink.

FOR THE STAGGERS.

DISSOLVE assafœtida in warm water, and put half a spoonful in each ear of the sheep—it is a speedy remedy.

TO PRESERVE FROM THE ROT.

TAKE the salt that is gathered from the marshes in summer, or for want of that, salt and alum; rub the mouth of the sheep with this once a week, and it will preserve them from the rot.

PART IV.

OF DISEASES IN SWINE.

A HOG is a very bad creature to doctor, therefore, to prevent their diseases, should be an object of our attention.

Keep him well, if you can, but not so as to burden him with fat in hot weather; keep his body open, and there will be little danger of his being sick. Brimstone, in small doses, is excellent for a hog; antimony is also good; but if you can get neither, chamber-lye put in their swill, will answer a good purpose. It is necessary to keep a hog's issues open; but I will make some remarks upon this elsewhere. The practice of feeding store hogs three times a day, is not good; whereas if they are fed only morning and night, they keep their appetite, eat their food clean, and grow the faster.

I shall now say a few things on the diseases of hogs.

MEASLES IN SWINE.

RUB them all over with a stiff brush dipped in cold water, then boil parsley roots and rue in salt water, and give it to them to drink.

FOR A FEVER.

LET them blood in the tail, and give them thrice a day water, wherein pepper and parsnip-roots have been boiled.

FOR THE SWINE POX.

TAKE an ounce of nitre, pound it, and disslove it in a pint of cider; add to it half a pint of sweet oil and one spoonful of honey, to be given to the swine luke warm.

FOR CATARRHS.

TAKE two ounces of coriander seed, one of ginger, three of honey, and half an ounce of turmeric, let it be powdered fine, and boiled in three quarts of new milk, then let the hog drink it.

OF DRENCHES.

IT is a practice among people in general, when their hogs are sick, to put a rope in their mouths and hang them up for drenching. This is a very bad practice—for while you are pouring your medicine down, the hog will squeak, and ten to one the liquid goes down the wind pipe and choaks him. If you can give your hog his medicine in milk, or some other liquid that he will drink, it is well; if not, do not force it down in the manner of drenching, but give it to him in the form of a clyster: This is always safe and as effectual as any method whatever.

ISSUES.

THE issues in a hog are places on the inside of their legs, which are porous, like a pepper box top. Here it seems, is the most immediate outlet for the superfluous fluid of the body: when these get stopped (as hogs are fond of filth and mire) the hog loses his appetite and becomes sick; then to drenching and choaking as before hinted; whereas, if his issues were rubbed and picked open, he would immediately recover.

Thus I have endeavoured in the preceding sheets, with much brevity and plainness, to treat upon those maladies, which have fallen more immediately under my inspection. I would not be thought a plagiary. I have made practical experience my guide, without regard to studied theories; I have not, however, discarded the sentiments of any man, because they agreed with my own; and if they may be in any measure serviceable to my readers, I shall never regret my trouble in writing them.

ADDITIONS.

Mr. JAMES SCAMMON'S RECEIPTS, OF STRATHAM.

To cure a Horse of the Bots.

Many horses die with the Bots, and often when people cannot tell what ails them; whereas, if the disorder was known, a cure might probably be effected. To know whether a horse has the Bots or not, first examine the inner part of the upper lip, and if you find several small bunches there, you may at once conclude he has the Bots.

Now, having got the disorder, we want a simple, safe, sure and easy remedy for their relief, which is as follows, providing they have not eat through the maw, viz.: Take one glass full of fine salt, and rub the bunches on the inner part of the lip with it until they all bleed, which causes the bots to break their hold on the maw; then give the horse potatoes plentifully for two or three days in succession, which loosens the horse and carries off the bots. I have often tried the experiment, and have never known it to fail of a cure.

A Cure for the Bots.

Take the entrails of a hen or chicken, and give them to a horse—it will cure him in a few hours. It may be done by raising the horse's head, opening his mouth, and putting them down his throat as far as you can, and he will swallow them.

A Cure for the Horn-ail in Cattle.

The cause of the Horn-ail is by a cold settling in the head, which stops or closes the pores or glands of the head, so that it does not have its natural discharge at the nose, which causes a collection of matter at the roots of the horns, and an inflammation through the body. The method of cure is as follows, viz.: First bore the horns; if they are hollow, put in some pork brine, with camphor and black pepper; then shear the hair off the head, between the horns; after which, mix one quart of salt with one pint of soap, and put it into a small bag made of thick linen or cotton and linen cloth, and confine it on the head between the horns; then bleed the creature, and take a discretionary quantity of blood according to the strength; two quarts from a creature that is strong or full blooded, and from a creature that is weak, one quart, once in three or four days, which seldom fails of having the desired effect of a cure. I have followed this method for several years, and I have not generally had occasion to dress their horns more than three or four times with the pork brine and camphor. I sometimes put a little vinegar into the nose to clear the head.

For disorders there is a natural cause, which requires reasonable means for its cure; therefore my reasons for the cure of the horn-ail are these: I use the pickle to clear the head, camphor and pepper to warm it, salt and soap to drive the inflammation into the body, and the bleeding to run it away.

To Cure a Horse of the Heaves.

The Heaves are generally caused by hard riding and sweating, and then letting the horse stand uncovered, thereby he takes one cold after another, until it settles so hard upon the lungs as to cause the heaves, which is similar to the asthma in a person, and it is generally thought to be incurable, therefore thousands of poor horses have to undergo the labour of the day while coughing and wheezing in a manner almost insupportable, only for the want of this simple remedy.—Take leaf tobacco and tie it on the bits of the bridle when the horse is used; likewise take one pound and a half of ginger for a horse; give two table spoonfulls a day, one in the morning and the other in the evening, mixed with wheat or rye bran, which seldom fails of curing the disease.

N. B. 'It takes the simple things of this world to confound the wise.'

A Cure for Cows and Oxen troubled with the Garget.

As soon as the cow's bag swells, or the milk curdles in the bag, or they give bloody milk, which is generally a sure indication of this disorder—First take two & a half quarts of blood from the creature; in three days after take away two quarts of blood, and in three days more take away one quart of blood, which is sufficient for the cure of any cow or ox whatever of the above disorder: but if owners of cows and oxen want to prevent their being troubled with this disease, I know of no better way than for them to bleed their cows about two weeks before the time of their calving, and their oxen in the spring, which I have known by experience to have prevented cows from having this disease for the whole season, notwithstanding they had before been blooded six or seven times in the course of a season, to keep them clear of this disorder, and prevent the loss of many quarts of milk.

N. B. By doing "a stitch in time may save nine," as the saying is.

For a Creature Choaked.

Take one cartridge of gun powder, and empty it down the throat of the creature as far as you can, by first drawing the tongue out, and when the tongue is drawn back, it will effect an immediate cure.

Cure for a Castrated Horse, or Sore Necked Ox, or Galled Horse.

Oint these, the above mentioned, with skunk's grease, dog's grease, or turtle's grease—if you please to use woodchuck's grease, it is much better—these will relieve the swellings.

For a Foundered Horse, by eating grain.

Pour spirits of turpentine into the frog of each hoof, holding it until it soaks in. This has cured when the horse was so stiff that he could not be led out of the stable. This was done immediately after the horse was injured.

Another for a Horse Foundered with grain.

Tanner's oil has been used to great advantage, by paring the hoofs very thin, and setting the shoes very close. Pour the oil inside of the shoe, and boil it in with a hot iron. This has been effectual.

For a Horse Foundered by drinking water.

Give him a glass of strong camphorated spirits. If done immediately, the first dose will give relief. If of a few days standing, the dose should be repeated a number of times.

It has been said by the experienced, that bleeding abundantly will give immediate relief in case of a founder by water or grain—half a pail full has sometimes been taken.

For Scouring of Cattle or Horses.

Use spirits of turpentine, by giving one spoonfull at a time. This has wrought great cures.

For the overflow in the Gall.

When a creature has the overflow in the gall he will lose his appetite; the white of his eye will be yellow. If you listen, you will discern a small hacking in his breath.

Cure—Take a hen's egg, pour out the white of it, fill it up equally with sut and salt; give a grown creature two of these in a day, to a smaller one, one in a day; thus continue till they are quite well. This has been used to very good effect. It is thought by some that the dose might be much larger.

Another for the overflow in the Gall.

A pint of soap and milk, equal in quantity, given three mornings or more, has been used to advantage.

For the Glands.

This disease is supposed to proceed from the relicks of the horse-ail not being properly physicked off. It is known also to proceed from a cold. The horse-ail is supposed to continue a fortnight or three weeks. This disease may be known by its longer continuance,—Its appearance is something similar, and may be cured, if its continuance has not been more than a year, and sometimes when it has been longer. Cure—Take white pine turpentine and garden colt's foot pulverized fine, mix them together and roll them into balls about the size of a hen's egg;

then take a skillet, fix a cover to it tight, bore an inch hole through the cover—turn a tin tunnel bottom upwards over it—put live coals into the skillet—place one ball thereon—hold the horse's nose over the tunnel snout one hour, and in this manner fumigate his head three times a day, and follow it three weeks, or longer if the appearance is favourable—and in some cases a cure has been wrought sooner.

A Bone Spavin comes by a bruise.
To cure it—take one ounce saltpetre, dissolve it in one quart of good rum, cork it up tight, and then rub it on; bathe it in every night and morning, if necessary—when first put on it causes more lameness. It is thought proper not to use the beast much.

Mr. ALLEN'S RECEIPTS, OF NEW-YORK.

Cure for Horses, for the Pool-evil and Thistalow.
Take the oil of vitriol, and drop a small quantity on the part affected, so repeat it till the pipes become clear; then carefully pull the pipe from the wound, wash it with cold water, and then oint it till it becomes sound.

Cure for the Heaves.
Take one pound of ginger, and half a pound of sulphur; mix them together, and give two ounces at a time for a dose in some kind of provender, once in two days.

To cure the Spavin.
Bathe it with the oil of origanum, with a small

quantity, once in two days; then take the oil of spike, and bathe it between the times above mentioned, with a hot shovel.

To cure the Scowers in Cattle or Horses.
Take a quantity of mullein, and boil it very strong—give from one to two quarts at a dose.

To Cure the Ring Bone.
Cut in the heel, after the fetlock, up and down, and then pull the bladder out, and oint the part affected. This bladder is caused by a weeping sinew.

For Ring Bones and Hard Spavins.
Oil of Vitriol, 1 oz. Spirits of Turpentine, 2 oz. Blubber Oil, 6 oz.

A table spoonful rubbed on every other day, and the next day rub with soap, and dry the medicine in with a hot brick. Take off the shoes and keep the hoofs dry, excepting greasing the hoofs.

N. B. Great caution ought to be used in mixing the oil of vitriol and spirits of turpentine, lest the effervescence burst the bottle; let the bottle therefore be uncorked to prevent danger.

Soft Spavins.
Take 3 oz. hog's fat—1 lb Indian-poke root—1 oz. spirits of turpentine, simmer them together over a moderate fire. Put on half a table spoonful every day, and rub it on the place affected.

For a Galled Horse.
To prevent white hairs coming out, grease the wound frequently.

To bring out hair where it refuses to grow, use the ashes of dead bees.

Proper conduct with Mares.

If there be any defect in your Seed Horse or Mares, as to their ancient blood, or as to any present disease, or ill form of any kind, it will affect the sprightliness, health and activity of your colts, allowing that your mares thus conceive. Choose horses as free from these defects as possible. It is thought proper for these horses, previous to their coming together, to be kept on clean oats and good old hay, for six weeks or a month at least. Let them come together in the morning fasting. If the mare is not ready, she may be courted by any other little horse that is sufficient for the purpose: let her be tied to a post, or stand perfectly in her own humour, without holding her up. When she is ready to receive the horse, let the horse be brought out to her with strong men on each side of him, to keep him orderly and straight forward till he leaps her. Let the cover be as natural and harmonious as possible. As soon as he is off, put on a pail of cold water; take the mare carefully away, and keep her from all horses, or the hearing of any, for three weeks, without her doing any labour. When she has taken the horse, let her not eat for four hours, nor drink till night, and let her food be as formerly, till the colt is well formed. After three weeks, let her be used carefully, without galloping her, without running her, without carrying heavy burdens on her back; without using her in very hot weather, and without sweating her; for either of these will cause her to cast her young. Be careful lest at any time she meets with a blow, or bruise, or strain, or wrench, or smells blood, at any time before she foals, lest she cast her young. When foaling, see that she is in a proper place, for a mare casts her foal standing. Let her keeper be present at the time of her foaling, and if the colt comes butt end first, let the hand be introduced into the body, and push the colt back, that he may come head first. And let her keeper as soon as she has licked her colt, milk her clean before the colt sucks, and stroke her several times; this will make her fruitful in giving milk, and prevent its curdling in her bag, so that she will not dry up. Some upon their mare's conceiving, have pared their hoofs very thin, and put on the hunters irons.

Moreover, if you are desirous to have your mare have a horse colt rather than a filly; observe then this lesson I shall here give you, and you will find it an infallible rule, and which shall never fail, viz.: At the time you would have your mare covered, let it be done when one of the five masculine signs do reign; which means when the sign is in the head, neck, arms, breast, or heart. But if she should be covered when any of the feminine or watery signs predominate; which means when the sign is in the belly, reins, secrets, thighs, knees, legs, or feet, then be you confident it will be a filly; for this I have often tried, and found it never to fail me, especially if the wind be west or north, (but west is the best) at the time of her covering, and you will find this, my rule, to be infallible, for experience hath taught me. After she has been thus covered, you shall know whether she hath conceived or cast her seed, by many evident symptoms which will appear to your eye; for if she containeth a good stomach for her meats, and so continueth—if she do not neigh at sight or hearing of other horses; if she do not piss often in the course of the day; casting not her eye about, gazing continually at every noise she heareth, pricketh not up her ears, and that in three or four days after her covering, her belly seemeth to be more gant, her hair more slick and close to her skin, and of a brighter colour, and she seemeth to fall away and become lean,—if, I say, any of these symptoms do appear in her, then it is an evident sign that she hath kept her seed and conceived; but if the contrary appear in her, then hath she lost it and gendereth not—but for her keeping and ordering after her covering, let her not drink what she desireth, but continue to her the same diet which she had formerly, for three weeks or a month.

To make the most valuable Green Horse Ointment.

Take a clean skillet, put in a piece of rosin the bigness of a walnut; when that is melted, put in a piece of wax the same bigness; when that is melted, put in half a pound of strained hog's fat; when that is melted, put in one spoonful of honey; when that is melted, stir all well together; then put in half a pound of turpentine; when this is melted, put in one ounce of verdigrise, ground very fine. If this causes a rising, set it off—when on again, stir in the verdigrise sufficiently, and let it simmer: but if it boils, it will turn red and lose its healing virtues, and be of a corrosive, hurtful nature. When it is simmered sufficiently, strain it into a clean earthen pot, cover it tight to preserve it from dust. If the grains are left in, it will be corrosive and prevent healing. This Green Ointment will cure all manner of chafes, bruises, or sores, especially if rubbed on every day and made to penetrate to the bottom of the sores. It will draw out splinters, stubs, nails, thorns, and is preferable to any other ointment whatever. It will keep flies and maggots from sores, and is very good for castrated horses: put it on when first castrated, and it will prevent swelling. Understanding Farriers, who have been acquainted with its healing virtues, have offered ten pounds to know how it was made. The copperas water is very good to be applied previous to the green ointment, to drench and wash the sore.

To make the valuable Copperas Water, to wash or syringe, or drench sores on Horses.

Take clean water 2 quarts, and put it into a clean pot, and put thereto of green copperas half a pound, salt one handful, honey one spoonful, and a branch or two of rosemary; boil all this till one half the water is consumed; and a little before you take it from the fire, put to it the quantity of a dove's egg of alum; then take it from the fire, and when it is cold, put the water into a glass, stop it up close, and keep it for your use; and when you are to dress any sore, first wash it clean with this water, and if the wound be deep, inject it with a syringe. This water of itself will cure any reasonable sore, or wound.

DR. DOW'S RECEIPTS, OF N. H.

For a Stoppage or Dry Belly Ache in a Horse or Ox.

The symptoms are a faltering, weakness, twisting and laying down. For relief, give one pint of Holland gin, and one half pint of molasses in the first stage of the disease—this has cured immediately. Let one person hold up his head by the under jaw, lay your hand edgewise across the creature's mouth, back of the fore teeth, and not pull out the tongue; put the neck of the bottle upon the top of the tongue, and let it run down under the edge of your hand.

To kill Bots in a Horse.

Take two ounces of alum, and the like quantity of dry hen's dung, pulverise these fine; put them into one pint of spirits, or any liquid; put it down the horse, and it will give immediate relief.

For the Bots.

Take one quart of blood from an ox, or any beef creature, and give it immediately while warm—this has been known to kill the bots immediately.

A cure for Ring Bones.

Boil what is called arsesmart into a good strong tea, wash the part with the liquor as hot as you can bear your hand in it, as often as twice or three times a day; if convenient wet a cloth in the liquor and bind it on the part after washing, and thus continue till quite well.

A cure for Wind Spavins, or Blood Spavins.

First bleed the horse in the leg below the gambril joint. For ointment, boil salt down to a brine as strong as possible; let it cool, take the scum that rises upon the top, one half a pint to one quarter of a pound of good tobacco, boiled as strong as possible in water, mixed with one quart of tea made strong of southern wood that grows in gardens—wash the part with these ingredients four or five times a day; bind on a cloth wet in the liquor; and they have been cured in three weeks. This liquor must be put on as hot as you can bear your hand in it. This also will cure bone spavins in the first stages of them. The horse must not be used while doctoring.

Mr. WHITTIER'S RECEIPTS, OF N. H.

For the Murrain in Cattle.

A quart of blood has been taken from the largest kind, and from the lesser in proportion. Fumigate their head with brimstone and old shoes, over a little fire, two or three times a day.

A cure for the Bots in Horses, if they have not got through the maw.

A quart of good dye stuff has given immediate relief.

For the Bots.

Half a pound of salts dissolved in warm water, has given immediate relief. There is one kind of bots that work in the great gut, close to the butt.

For a stoppage or Dry Belly Ache in a Horse.

Take a pot that holds a pail full and a half, or more—pack it full of clover hay and water—boil it down to two or three quarts, and pour it down the horse—it will physic through him, and give immediate relief.

For a stoppage in the manifold of a neat creature.

It generally proceeds from strains, taking cold, and low keeping, which causes the wind to stop, and the creature loses his appetite, swells moderately, and has a rattling in his throat more than they have with the overflowing of the gall. Cure,

Take one pint of hog's fat, one pint of molasses, and one pint of mustard seed ground fine; mix these all together; give them to the creature blood warm—wait three hours, and if there is no movement, give from a half a pound to a pound of salts put in warm water, according to the constitution and disorder of the creature. After waiting a proper time, repeat the salts if needed.

The symptoms of the Water Garget,

Are sinking eyes, of a yellow cast, dry nose—often if the side is stroked, it will rattle like parchment. Cure—Take from a common creature a pint and a half of blood; then measure a pint of smart weed and a pint of hoarhound, by pressing each into a pint dish tight; simmer these two pints, and get the tea out well, and give this to the creature. Repeat this dose three mornings. This we have not known to fail.

The symptoms of the Yellow garget,

Is the loss of the cud, from the stomach being too weak to raise; the lights are full of filthy, frothy matter—the joints are quite weak. Cure, Take half a pint of garget root, and half a pint of garlicks, boil these in a quart of new milk; give this to them ealy in the morning for three mornings—we always find it to be a cure.

For the Castration of Horses.

Let the sign be in the feet or legs, or thereabouts. When you cut him, do not strain the string, but take a piece of twine and tie the middle of the twine round a piece of salt pork, an inch long, and half an inch wide, and tie this round the string of the horse, half an inch above where you cut off the stone, and then cut off the string close to the stone; then bathe all his secret parts with lamp oil. In this way we have not known them to swell, nor any evil to follow.

For the Staggers in Horses.

Half a pint of rum and a spoonful of powder, ground fine, and given to a horse, has relieved frequently.

To cure Oxen poisoned by eating Kill Lamb.

Three oxen were poisoned among us by eating kill lamb (called by some, lorrel); they were so bad that they reeled and staggered, and were likely to have died, had not something been done. They gave them one pint of rum; in a few hours they began to amend, and in a few days they got entirely well.

There is a bush that is ever green, called spoonhunt; this poisons sheep, and it is likely it would cattle, if they ate it. A cow was poisoned by the above lorrel; they gave her half a pint of rum, and she got well.

To cure a Horse of the Canker.

A young man among us, who had a young horse six years of age, that had the canker in his mouth, round about his jaw and on his tongue. The cankery spots were whitish, and appeared like common eating canker. There was information obtained from the Farriers. The direction of one was, to rub his mouth with alum pounded fine, once in a while, and bleed him. The direction of the other was, to bleed him, and wind a good wisp of wild willow bark (off the root—it is redish) about his bits, tieing it tight at each end of the bits—riding him with the bits thus fixed. Let the horse stand in the barn with the bits in, as much as you can. The young man used the bark only, and in a few days his horse got well.

For the Gripes.

A man amongst us had a horse of some age, that was taken rolling, tumbling and striving, as though he would die, till at length he laid still. His master mixed half a pint of rum with half a pint of molasses, and stirred in half a pint of milk, put it into a junk bottle, and went to the horse, raised up his head, put the snout of the bottle into his mouth, and turned it down without resistance. In less than an hour the horse was well. This medicine is good for the bots.

To stop a horse from bleeding in the nose, or elsewhere.

Take the tender tops of hyssop and jam them up, put them into his nose, or lay and bind them on the wound, and the blood will be stopped.

To cure the Barbs in horses.

There is a disease in horses called the barbs. It groweth under the tongue, for every horse hath them. Nevertheless, there is no harm in them till they become inflamed with humour and bad blood—then they will swell and trouble the horse so that he cannot eat without much sorrow. Cure—Take hold of his tongue and pull it out, and underneath, on either side by the jaws, you will see two teats or little breasts; clip or cut them away, and wash the place with salt and water, and they will get well. Be careful that hay chaff does not get in and prevent their healing.

For the Bots in Horses.

It is said that poplar bark and white ash bark, pulverized and mixed with provender and given to horses, will cure the bots.

Another for the Bots.

When they trouble a horse they may be driven back with spirits of turpentine; or they may be struck off the maw with your fist by striking smartly a number of times: the horse will show where they are. Then make a tea of a bunch of hemlock boughs as big as you would have for a broom. Strain the tea and put into it one quart of rye; then boil them sufficiently long for the tea to soak into the rye. Give this to the horse immediately after the bots have been drove back. Give him the like dose three times in the course of one or two days. It is said to be an effectual remedy.

Another for the Bots.

Either bleed the horse in the mouth so that he may swallow a pint of blood, or give him three pints of sweetened milk; after you have done one of these, wait an hour, then give him half a pint of flax-seed oil; after a short time give him another half pint of the oil.

Another for the Bots or Worms.

Take a tumbler full of savine boughs, cut fine, mix them with meal, or his provender when you give it to him.

Another remedy for the Bots.

A strong decoction of dogwood, sometimes

called poison sumach, is excellent for the bots or worms.

Another for the Bots.

When you cannot get the other things mentioned for the bots, you may use spirits of turpentine and rum mixed together—a gill of each is thought to be sufficient, as it gives great pain, and if the horse is feeble, it is likely he will not stand it. Put it down the horse. If you are afraid the bots will kill the horse before you can do any thing to purpose, rub a little spirits of turpentine on his breast as near the maw as possible; a little on his chops, if you please, and it will drive them back.

For the Heaves.

A small quantity of assafœtida, dissolved, put in his provender a number of times, and a little wound about his bits, has cured. Tobacco has been used in the same manner.

For the Heaves—a difficulty from the wind being hurt.

Take hornets nests, comb and all, pick it into pieces and mix it with his provender; immediately after this, give him some boiled potatoes. This will relieve when the horse is very bad. Give it to him before using him. If you boil the provender and nest together, the horse will eat it much better.

A description of Savine and Cedar.

White cedar grows in swamps, savine and red cedar grows on upland. The white cedar has a rough seed coming out near the end of the twigs. Savine has a seed growing out near the end of the twigs which is smoother than that of the white cedar—they appear the last of May. The burrs of white cedar hang all winter. White cedar has flat plaidish boughs, its limbs are white clear through.

The red cedar and savine on upland;—their difference may be known by their limbs. The savine limbs are white clear through, but the inside of the red cedar limbs are dark crimson. There are juniper trees much like the savine; the plums are smaller and the bough not so bitter.

For the Castration of any creature.

This ought to be done when the sign is in the feet or legs. When this is done, do not strain the string, but cut it off as near the stone as you can. Take spirits of turpentine and pour into each hole, one tea spoonful for a young creature, and a table spoonful for a bullock; hold it together a little while, and it will prevent bleeding. If a horse, let him be seared. If they swell, use dog's grease, or skunk's grease—woodchuck's grease is better. The contrary practice on these creatures is much worse to heal, and destroys their strength, courage and toughness to a great degree.

To cause a horse to vomit.

Take two great roots of poly-podium off the oak—it is said to grow on rocks—scrape it clean, and tie it to the bits, and when steeped in the oil of spike a whole night, then in the morning, fasting, put on his bridle with the roots fastened to his bits, and ride him softly for an hour or more— if he be troubled with any rheumatic, phlematic humour, or cold, which may clogg or annoy his stomach. It will cause him to vent or vomit at his mouth or nose, and to cough, sneeze and send forth a great quantity of filth and slimy matter; and in a short time he becomes very clean in his body; for this will both refine his blood and exhaust all the watery humours in such a manner, as by temperate usage, and doing as here prescribed, you may keep him a long time sound. You may give it to a horse newly taken from grass, or to any horse that has taken a cold. Some have given white wine and honey afterwards to nourish the blood.

To keep flies from tormenting a horse.

Take the leaves of gourds, pumpkins or cucumbers, stamp or pound them, and strain them, and with the juice thereof wash your horse all over, and the flies will not come near him. This has been often proved.

Another.—Take mallows, stamp or pound them, and strain them, and with the juice thereof wash your horse, and it will keep away the flies. This is an approved good thing.

Another.—Take verdigrise, ground very fine, boil it in vinegar, and wash him therewith, being careful that none gets into his eyes or ears. This is the best and will last the longest.

For a disease in horses called the Flying Worm, Tetter, or Ring Worm.

This is a humour appearing under the hair. Cure—Take of precipitate 2 drachms, and put it into a small viol with spring or good running water, much more than will cover the powder, keeping it close stopped; and with this water wash the place once every day, and it will sure-

F

ly effect a cure. When you have used this water, stop it up close, and shake it together—dress it twice a day.

For a horse gravelled.

Search and find the gravel, then stop the place with hog's grease and turpentine, mixed together; pour it in scalding hot; stop it up with hurds; then tack on the shoe, keep his feet from wet, and he soon will be well.

To cure a horse of the Flux or Scowers.

Take the entrails of a young hen, or a great chicken, excepting the gizzard; mix one ounce of spikenard with them, and make him swallow it; this will infallibly stay his scouring; yea, if it be a bloody flux, this is very good.

Treatment of Horses, &c.

Pulse of a Horse.—In the management of sick horses great advantage may be derived from attending to the state of the pulse, as we are thereby enabled to judge of the degree or violence of the disease, and the probability there may be of recovery. We are in some measure also assisted by it in ascertaining the nature of the complaint, and the application of remedies.

In a healthy horse the pulsations are about 36 or 40 in a minute, and may be felt very distinctly either on the left side, or in an artery which passes over the lower jaw bone; in short, pulsation may be felt in every superficial artery.

When a horse appears rather dull and does not feel properly, it is advisable to examine the pulse, & if he be found to exceed the standard of health, immediate recourse should be had to bleeding. By this timely inteference many dangerous complaints may be prevented. When the pulse rises to 80 in a minute, there is reason to be apprehensive of danger; and when it exceeds 100 the disease frequently terminates in death.—*White's Treatise.*

Do not get your horse too warm. If he drinks when he is quite warm, hold up his head every two or three swallows. If he drinks much when he is very warm, ride him smartly, to warm it in his belly—it may prevent hurting him.

When you use your horse with the saddle, examine his back every night; if it swells, take a handful of his wet litter and lay it on, and put his saddle on over it for one night; it will cure it by the morning.

If your horse's back is chafed raw, lay on burdock leaves under the saddle—it is good to heal. But if you are obliged to use your horse in this chafed condition, pound up toad plantain, and lay it on the sore when you tackle, every morning; this will toughen the sore, and has cured when nothing else would.

When you bleed in the mouth, Farriers say it is best in the third wrinkle. If you cannot stop the blood, ride him smartly a quarter of a mile or more, and this will stop it. If by bleeding in the neck you cut through the vein, so that he swells by the blood under the vein, bathe it liberally with cold water, and it will cure him. For a horse foundered bleed him well in the feet; it is thought to be the surest remedy.

If you heat your horse too much, it will melt his grease, and cause it to run down into his legs, and make him disordered there and elsewhere, in a grievous manner.

When a horse drops his water straight down, it indicates that he has been strained across his back or kidneys, and oftentimes hurts him, especially when low in flesh.

A horse strained at the short joint below the gambrel, will throw his foot out as he takes it up. A horse that is spavined at the gambrel joint, will take his foot right up, as though he would keep it up too much.

At the first appearance of scratches on horses, rub on the grease that comes from the top of the pot, warm a few times, and there is not much danger.

Rye, unless boiled, is apt to make horses weak in the joints.

MEDICAL RECEIPTS.

For a Child that is stuffed up.

Take goose oil, or olive oil, rub it up and down on each side of the nose, and round about the eyes. If the child is pressed at the stomach, take a portion of the goose oil, enough to puke it. If the child's difficulty appears to be that of the rattles, or is some like the quincy, take a great spoonful of goose grease and two spoonfuls of chamber lie, (and in the same proportion for a larger quantity) and mix them by warming them on embers, and sweeten it with a spoonful of honey, if you can get it, if not, with molasses, and give it to the child forcibly and sufficiently, pausing now and then to prevent the child's strangling to death. This has caused them to strive and puke up the bladders, whereby the child was relieved. Repeat it if necessary.

For Corns on the Feet.

Take apple-perue leaves, jam them and rub them on; or you may simmer them down strong in a spoonful of hog's fat, and oint the corns therewith, or bind it on.

To cure the Asthma.

Take the bag that holds the musk of a skunk, and hang it up in the room where the person lives—rub it about the mouth and nose, smelling of it often—if very bad, take two or three drops of the musk, or more, as you need. This has given great relief, so that the speechless have been relieved, and have got well.

For the Cramp Rheumatism.

Take 25 or 30 drops of the spirits of turpentine on sugar every morning for three weeks, and it will cure said rheumatism.

For the Ague in the face.

Take smart weed and jam it up well, wet it with rum and bind it on, or you may boil it and lay it on.

For the Wind Cholic.

Take one large puff ball, or two or three small ones, boil them in a pint of skimmed milk for half an hour; take one half at a time. When seized in a less degree, in a hypochondriacal way, scalded skimmed milk, taken hot, frequently, is very good.

For the Dysentery.

Take black cherries, put them into rum, make the rum quite strong with them. You may prepare them by pounding them up, dry or green, seeds and all. Give to the patient as much as he can bear. Clear him out with physic first, if the dysentery has not done it. Castor oil is good physic.

A Receipt for that disease which is properly called a stoppage in the water.

Take one pint of black ash kees, (these come out in September) boil these in one gallon of water to one quart, add one quart of Holland gin—take of this half a glass night and morning.

Another receipt for the stoppage in water.

Take from ten to fifteen drops of balsam copaiva night and morning. This difficulty arises from a stricture or weakness in that part.

Spirits of turpentine has been used for this difficulty to good advantage. Take one tea spoon full night and morning, or less, if it operates too severely.

A pill made of white pine turpentine the bigness of a pea, taken night and morning, has cured this difficulty when medical skill has failed.

To prevent Fits.

Deer's horn rasped fine, and made into a tea, has been given to great advantage.

Spikenard pounded fine and mixed with sharp vinegar, & made warm, is an excellent application for a bruise of the side, or any other part of the body.

For the Dysentery.

In cases of long standing, and when the inflammatory symptoms have subsided, give ten drops of spirits of turpentine, dropped on to a little sugar two or three times a day—for children a less quantity.

A receipt to kill Corns.

Take three cents, put them into a tea cup with good strong vinegar, enough to cover them, let it set a week or fortnight, or until it is considerably dried away, so as to become thickish, then dip a little rag in it, and bind it on the corns several times.

To take a Film off the Eye.

Drop in the juice of wild celandine, (called by

some wild sulindine) if this is too smart for the eye, mix it with breast milk, and it will take off the film from the eye; it is also good for cloudiness. Loaf sugar pounded up fine and put into the eye, has taken away the film in the first stages of it. The above mentioned herb simmered down to a salve or oil, and put into the eye, answers a good purpose. The use of this herb, as above mentioned, has restored the eye sight when it had failed for many years.

For Sore Eyes.

Use the juice of wild celandine, by putting it frequently in the eyes—it has restored the eyes when very bad, and of long standing.

Symptoms of the Maw Worm,

Is paleness of face, and whitishness about the mouth, and uneasy feelings. The maw worm is small, about half an inch long, and very numerous, and trouble children and persons of age. A child has been cured by eating frequently of all kinds of beans, baked or stewed together with pork. This was continued for two weeks, in which time the worms passed off very numerously. The child craved the beans. This worm is not like the other kind of little flat stomach worms, or large worms; it inhabits the maw or ponch.

For a Scald or Burn.

Lay on a linen cloth wet with rum for twelve hours—then at night lay on a linen cloth spread over with hog's fat, grated over with the red ross of a large hemlock—put this on every night, and put on the cloth wet with rum every day, washing it at intervals with a tea made of white pine bark—and put on a little goose grease a few times when you have washed it in rum. This has cured a child in four or five weeks that was scalded down her neck and each side of her shoulder for half a foot. It was said to be a very bad scald.

A Plaster for a Pain in the back, or in the Side.

Take some pitch from white pines that have been slivered about a year—spread a plaster on soft leather; then powder camphor, and strew it on the top of the pitch, and strew on as much sulphur.

For a Pain in the Stomach, or for the Bilious Cholic, or any other Cholic, and for the wind in the Stomach.

Take ginson root, (this is more properly called Bath root) a piece as big as from the end to the joint of your little finger for a child, and for older persons accordingly--grate it fine, and steep it in water, and drink it as warm as you can. After pausing a little while, if it does not relieve, give more in quantity. It is said by physicians that it operates like laudanum on the human frame. For the above complaints it has been found to cure when nothing else would.

For the Jaundice complaint in persons, or the overflow of the gall in creatures.

Take white ash bark off the root, and poplar bark off the root, and black cherry tree bark from the body of the tree, in equal quantities—steep them well—put the tea with cider, and drink of it morning, noon and night, a tumbler full for a person as long as he needs it—and a quart for a creature, and repeat it until it physics his difficulty away. When they have this disorder, they will hang their head and will not eat, and the white of the eye is yellowish.

To cure the Sore Throat.

Take red succory, make a good tea of it, and drink a tea cup full of it at night, when you go to bed—smoke a piece of the stalk, by setting one end of it on fire, at bed time.

Cure for Fever and Ague.

One handful of horsemint, 4 oz. of shee or tall mullen root scraped fine, 4 oz. ginson or stink weed root scraped fine, 3 red pepper pods, the whole to be boiled in 3 quarts of water down to 3 half pints; then strained and sweetened—one half to be taken at the first symptom of the shake, as hot as possible, the other half to be taken in half an hour.

For the King's Evil.

Take poke stalks and leaves, fry them in a clean frying pan, or spider, and it will become liquid. Rub it on the king's evil sufficiently for a number of times, or bind on a cloth wet with the liquor. Cork it in a bottle if you have need to keep it.

Another for the King's Evil.

Take the oldest leaves under a chesnut tree, and steep them in water, wash the sore with the liquor, and bind the leaves on the sore; after this take some salts to physic the blood.

A cure for the Asthma.

Take and dissolve saltpetre in water, so strong that it will stand in the bottom of a bottle—take brown paper enough for a good segar, wet it thoroughly in this petrified water; then dry it three quarters dry, and roll it into a segar; then burn it in the room where the distressed person is—close the room tight, and in thirty minutes he will rest perfectly easy.

A good and wholesome physick for those that need.

Take a small handful of butternut bark, (some call it oil nut) simmer it to a strong tea; give the person one glass, then wait an hour, and if there is no operation, give half a glass; wait half an hour; if there is no movement, give one spoonful, and so continue every half hour until it operates.

To cure hard drinking.

Take Roman wormwood, gather it in the full of the moon when it is in the blossom, and in the morning when the dew is on; dry it one day in the sun, then under cover until it is dry, roll it up in paper, then put it into a tight place, and make a bitter of this by putting it into water—drink this frequently, and when you are faint—so continue one year, and it will deliver you from the desire of ardent spirit. This is called Roman wormwood, because it cured the Romans of a stinking breath.

Another cure for drinking ardent spirits.

When you feel faint, and feel as though you want some spirit, drink water, and it will relieve your faintness, and cure your desire for ardent spirits; whereas the contrary practice causes the fibers and tendons to be ossified, and the inside to be of a seared and decaying nature, which increases your thirst for spirit, and destroys your health and wealth. It has a great operation on the liver, and oftentimes makes it hard & seared.

For the Asthma and Cough—this is a cure even if it has been of long standing.

Cure—Snakeweed, more properly called bastort—take one gill & a half of the leaves, & put them into one quart of new rum—take half a wine glass of this, and sweeten it with half a spoonful of molasses, and stir it well together—take this portion every morning, half an hour before breakfast. This will cleanse the head and stomach well of catarrh, or any other disorder. It will do to put one quart of rum to this steep the second time. This steep has cured the cough and asthma of more than twenty years standing. One half a drachm of the root, pulverised, is supposed to be stronger than the steep above mentioned.

For an inflamed, feverish, swelled Leg.

Take the inside of basswood bark, scrape it fine, and pour hot water on to it, for a poultice; lay this on to still the pain. The bark off the root, pounded fine, and simmered with skimmed milk, will bring down the swelling much better, if it does not stick too much.

To kill Worms in Children.

Take sage, boil it with milk to a good tea, turn it to whey with alum or vinegar, and give the whey to the child, if the worms are not knotted in the stomach, and it will be a sure cure. If the worms are knotted in the stomach, it will kill the child.

For Worms.

Make a fine powder of black or spotted alder bark, that bears the red plumb, scraping the bark down—give it to the child in molasses, or any thing handy. This has cured when the skill of the physician failed.

For Sore Eyes.

When your eyes begin to be sore, wash them in cider a few times, night and morning. This has cured.

For Consumptive Complaints.

For a person that has strained his stomach, and has other consumptive complaints; or for a person that has consumptive complaints without this sprain, such as the following, viz. pain in the stomach or side, headache, and often attended with cough. Cure—Make one quart of good tea of the herb called vervine, by boiling it in cider, strain it and bottle it up, and take a glass night and morning, or less as you are able—repeat this quantity as long as it helps you. There are two kinds of vervine, blue and white; use the blue for women, and the white for men, if you can get them, if not, use the kind or kinds you can get. This has relieved the youth and aged, and has been used by an approved physician in Portsmouth.

For a humour in the Leg by a hurt or strain.

There was a man amongst us about sixty years of age, that travelled in the snow and strained his leg, by which the humour settled, and in a little while it was useless. The doctor of the town attended it without success; and there was a doctor consulted in an adjacent town, of uncommon information. His direction was, go to a spring and get frogs sufficient to cover his leg, when they were baked well in brandy in an earthen pot so as to stir them up like a thin

G

pudding, spread it on a woollen cloth sufficient to cover his leg, and bind it on his leg—he was commanded to wear it several days, while the bones pricked him—he thus did and his leg was soon restored, and was as well as the other.

For the Ague Fever.—Men have it sometimes when they come from sea.

Take a junk bottle and fill it with his urine, just as the shake is coming on; cork it tight and bury it two feet deep. This has given entire relief in this difficulty. Whether it would operate thus in the fever ague, I cannot say.

For Sore Eyes.

The inside of sassafrass soaked in cold spring water, and rubbed on the eyes a few times, has been known to cure.

For the Dysentery.

A tea made of frost weed root, more properly called coak ash root, and drank freely, has given great relief.

For an inward Fever.

Take one bunch of spleen roots, pound them up and steep them in cool water—drink of the tea several times in the course of a day—it is said to be good.

Hog-tush brake root, steeped in warm water, without boiling—when it is cool, take it for the above complaint.

For the Dysentery.

Take the suet of mutton, slice it, and simmer it over the fire slowly—when dissolved, take two spoonfuls once in two hours. Take poped or parched corn, soak it in sweet milk, eat the corn and drink the milk with no other food.

Cure for Cold.

Take half a pound of raisins, one gill of flaxseed,

two ounces stick lickorish, put the same into 4 quarts of water, and boil it down one half; strain and sweeten it with half a pound of loaf sugar.

Cure for Consumption.

Take half a pound of spikenard, one pound of cumfrey, half a pound of elecampane, put them into four quarts of water, and boil it down one half—strain it, and add one pound of loaf sugar.

Worm Pills.

Take butternut buds in the spring of the year, dry them and grind them to powder, make the powder into pills of the bigness of a small pea, and take one when going to bed at night.

Cure for puking up food.

Take an old pipe, and powder the same—take from half to a teaspoonful on an empty stomach in the morning.

Cure for a bad Cough.

Take of loaf sugar, sweet oil and spirits of hartshorn, an equal quantity, and mix them together about the thickness of honey; take a teaspoonful when the cough is troublesome.

To make a Plaster to be put on the bottom of the feet, when the head is pressed with hypocondriack and humour.

Take a potion of tar, and a little more turpentine than tar, warm these on the fire and mix them, and thicken it up with ginger, sufficient for a plaster, and lay it on to the bottom of the feet, as large as you conveniently can, and let it remain as long as it will stick, (it may be three weeks) and repeat it.

To cure the Toothache.

Put one ounce of alum and one ounce of sweet nitre into a viol together—drop in a drop or too into the hollow of the tooth, now and then, and it will kill the tooth and prevent its aching better than to pull it. This is the opinion of the doctors.

For Children when they have Worms and the Worm Fever.

Take little snake weed, and make a tea of it, and give it to them frequently—it will destroy the worms and cure the fever.

This herb appears with a small white blow the first of May—the latter part of May the blow disappears, and early in the season the herb disappears also.

For the Rheumatism in the Cords, Muscles or Joints.

Cure—Take hog's pissle grease one gill, beef's gall half a glass, spirits of turpentine one ounce, simmer them together, then add one gill of Cognac brandy. Use—when it is cold, warm and mix it, and bathe the affected part at night. The above is good for bruises and sprains. In rheumatism it generally relieves in about a week.

A sovereign remedy for the Jaundice.

Babary bark off the root, barberry bark off the stock, and meadow parsley, (sometimes called golden thread) an equal proportion of these to the amount of a tea-cup full in the whole, pounded fine, then take three pints of water from a living spring, boil it down to one pint, put it to a pint of rum, and put in the powders; cork it up in a bottle; take one glass, more or less, as you are able to bear. Take it in the morning and at one o'clock.

For the Catarrh.

The root of Hellebore, sometimes called Indian poke, pounded fine and sifted, and taken in snuff, provokes to sneezing in a very powerful manner, and is good for the catarrh. It has relieved from craziness when the brain is pressed by a stoppage.

For the Piles.

Take Canada thistle roots and simmer them in cream, then take a linen rag two inches square, wet it with the ointment thus simmered, twist it and put it up the bowel. This has wrought a cure in three days—repeat it every day.

For the Cancer or Scrofula Humour.

Take a pail full of pyrola umbrellata, (or as it is called noble pine, and by the Westerns pipsissewa) add three pails of water, boil the same 6 hours, strain off the liquor, and boil the same down to three quarts; pour that hot upon 1 lb. of sulphur in a new gallon stone jug, shake the same for 30 minutes, then add 1 quart of Holland gin, cork the same up, and take from a table spoon full to a glass, as the patient can bear, four or six times a day, and apply the same as a wash to the tumour.

For inward Humour or Rheumatism.

Garget berries or roots, sliced fine, and put in spirits, has often effected a wonderful cure.

To heal an Old Sore.

Wild valerian leaves, or honey, have healed when the case was difficult.

For Cough or Cold.

Take tea made of hoarhound, one teacup full night and morning. This frequently relieves.

For the Canker.

Take 2 or 3 red peppers, make a strong tea of them and give it to the person. This, though harsh, will relieve in fifteen minutes, wonderfully.

For a Cold.

Take the vines of five-finger, make a good tea of it, and give to the person frequently.

For the Dysentery.

Make a good tea of five-finger vines and roots, and give it frequently to the person.

For a Fever.

Make a good tea of five-finger roots, and give it sufficiently to the person. This has been known to cure a fever after a person has had it four or five days.

For a Cough.

Take witchwood bark, and make a good tea of it—take a teaspoonful at going to bed and in the morning for about three days, or longer if necessary.

Elecampane is good to loosen a cough—take a piece as large as a common white bean.

For a Green Wound, or Cut.

Make a tent of linen lint, and wet it in spirits of turpentine and lay it into the wound, and there let it be until it heals—by wetting it with a feather dipped in the same spirits, morning and evening.

For the Dropsy.

A tea of dwarf elder root, continually drank, has cured the dropsy.

To kill Ringworms.

Take a little spirit in a spoon, and put a teaspoonful of gun powder into it, rub it up fine with the finger, and rub it on, and it scarcely ever fails of curing it the first time it is put on. The juice of wild celendine rubbed on repeatedly will also cure: this juice will also cure other cankerous humours. The oil of red corn pressed out between hot irons and rubbed on several times, will also cure the ringworm.

Dr. John Smith's receipt for curing the Toothache.

Take the bark of white oak, the bark of babary root, the root of elecampane, and the root of winter green, of each an equal quantity—boil them over a slow fire until the strength is out; then add one half pint of black pismires, baked in an oven in an earthen pot, covered over with a crust of doe; then add this with the other; boil them down to half a pint, stir in some flour, and make it into pills suitable for the hollow in the tooth—apply this for four or five times, and it will effect a cure.

The four first mentioned have proved a cure, by holding the liquor in the mouth until the strength is out, three or four times, as hot as you can bear it.

Elecampane root grated and made into a pill and applied to the hole in the tooth, has relieved the pain a little.

Mr Daniel Tenney's receipt to cure Sore Eyes.

Take one teaspoonful of white vitriol to two spoonfuls of water, or mix in that proportion; wet the eyes with the same at night, and rub it in with the end of your finger every night, and oftener if you please, and thus continue until they get well. The operation will be sharp but without damage, & the cure will soon be wrought.

To cure a Felon or Whitlow before it is ulcerated.

Take the skin out of a good hen's egg, and put it on the felon, and keep it on until your are relieved of the pain.

For a weak Stomach, and Consumptive Complaints.

Take balsam copayva, and drop five or six drops on sugar, or more, if you think proper.

The best Plaster for weakness, or pain in the back.

Is to take balsam from the cracked or bruised part of the hemlock tree—prepare a plaster of it the bigness of your hand, by warming by the fire, not heating it—spread it thinish. If it blisters so that the plaster comes off, you may make it stick again by warming it, and the effect will be very good.

To cure Corns.

Mix pulverized chalk with soap, sufficient for a salve to spread into a plaster, and bind it on the corn two or three times, or more, if needed.

For a Cough.

Make a candy by boiling down hoarhound in molasses—Take a piece as big as a walnut, night and morning, or more, if you think proper.

For Fevers.

The soldiers in the late war, at Burlington, were visited with the putrid nervous fever (it is called the typhus) and many of them were taken away. Many things were tried without effect to cure them; at length a large trough was prepared and filled with hemlock tea made of the boughs. The languishing, when put into this bath for thirty minutes, or more, were recovered without any relapse or ill effects.

When the spotted fever was about, one man gave command to lay on mullen leaves wet in warm water all over him, with the upper side to him, which is drawing, the other side is driving. Thus they did, although he was struck senseless, and he was cured.

Another man with the same fever, ordered, to take a bushel of salt, one half of it to be laid on a woollen blanket under him; the other half spread over him, and covered up with woollen cloths. They thus did, & he was cured.

For the Relax and Dysentery—by James Scammon.

Take allspice 1 spoonful, salt 1 spoonful, pulverize these fine, put an egg with them, & beat them up well; mix this with half a pint of milk, and take it. Take the like dose once an hour till well.

For the Dysentery.

Eat the fat of mutton, or take it fried out, or any way you can get it down. The fat off the kidney is best. This is very excellent.

For the Canker.

It is thought by some that cooling things should be given, but by the experienced, it is well known that hot things produce a valuable effect, as the canker comes by colds.—A glass of strong tea made of red pepper, and given to the person, has relieved the mouth and throat greatly in fifteen minutes.

For Burns, to prevent blistering.

Spirits of turpentine and cotton wool, applied immediately, will prevent blistering.

A Cure for Corns.

Take houseleek, jam it up and bind it on.

For the Dropsy.

Take off the large milkweed tops and leaves, when green, make a strong tea of them—to every teacup full add a spoonful of best Holland gin. Dose—a teacup full every one or two hours, as may suit the stomach. N. B. The gin to be added when you take the dose. The roots of milkweed will answer the same purpose.

For the Dysentery.

Take the root of cattail flag, peal off the outside bark, and pick it to pieces, put milk with it, and boil it to a palp—drink it, and eat it, and live upon it.

For the Rheumatism.

Take garget berries and put a sufficient quantity in one quart of rum, and take one glass at a time. They have been put in brandy sometimes.

For a Cut, to prevent soreness.

Take spleen roots, jam them up and put them on the wound for a poultice; it will prevent soreness, or take out soreness. Hog-tush brake root will answer the same.

For the Fever and Ague.

Take a handful of culver's root, put it into one quart of rum, and take three glasses a day, if you can bear it. There are two kinds of this root; it grows two feet or more high, and has leaves at each joint, one bearing a blue blossom, the other white. The difference here mentioned, may be termed a dark or light crimson.

For the Dysentery.

Take one spoonful of whiskey, and one spoonful of wheat flour, mix these together, and take the like dose once an hour for four of five times.

A Receipt for the Canker.

Take swamp willow bark off the root (it is redish) mix it with rattle-snake-bite; get the tea out of them. Give it to the person every five minutes, if bad. Make a strong tea of the bark to cleanse the mouth, previous to taking the other tea. A rag wet in the first tea is good for any cankerous sore. Make a powder of the same bark if a person cannot take the tea.

For a Cough.

Take hemlock boughs and fill a pail pot with boughs and water closely packed—boil them nearly three hours—then take out the boughs, strain the water, and cleanse the pot. Boil the liquor down to half a pint. Cork it in a bottle—take a tea spoon full at a time three times a day, and thus continue unless it sinks your spirits too much.

Receipt for the Rheumatism.

Take arse-smart weed, boil it in water, and drink it freely. Likewise, make a linen bag about eight inches long—fill it with the above weed and boil it in a pint of W. I. Rum until it becomes strong. Apply it below the pit of the stomach as warm as can be borne. Keep renewing it until the pain subsides.

For Deafness.

Take a little bunch of sage, wrap it up in rye dough, bake it in the oven, not too hard; pick a little hole open against the sage, and by means of this, press the steam into the ear.

Another for Deafness.

Take a green black ash stick of wood, lay it on the fire, when the juice comes out catch it in something that is clean. Cork it in a vial. Drop two drops at a time into the ear, twice a day or oftener. If you go out and take cold, it will prevent its good effect.

Pickerel's oil dropped into the ear, has been used to good purpose.

Cure for Worms, or any person whose Victuals hurt them.

Take a piece of deer's horn an inch long; burn it to a coal and pulverize it fine, or you may saw the same quantity to sawdust; mix these with molasses or any other liquid, or you may prepare it by whittling and pounding it fine and getting the tea out. It may be given in either of these three ways.

To cure a Felon after it is Ulcerated.

Roast an onion until the rind comes off. Bind it on the felon as hot as you can get it. Roast the remainder of the onion until another rind comes off. Apply it as before, and so continue until the pain subsides.

To cure a Felon.

Take a quart of skimmed milk, skim'd clean, put three gills of water with it, and one handful of salt in it, then set it on fire coals, and when it begins to simmer, put in your finger, or felon, and keep it in while it boils; dont take it out till it boils, lest it strike to your stomach. This will give immediate relief and a safe cure.

To cure a Whitlow or Burn.

Take the skin of hog's suet and bind it on two or three times; if the whitlow breaks out, bind it on till it gets well—the effect is excellent.

Dr. Morse's receipt to draw a Felon to a head.

Boil flaxseed in new milk, and at the last stir in some Indian flour. Repeat this poultice so often as to keep it warm, and it will speedily draw it to a head.

To harden or help your fingers when they are cracked by drawing a thread through them.

Take the oil of corn, pressed out between hot irons, rub it on the cracked places, warming it in by the fire.

For Cracked, or Sore Lips.

Use the oil of walnut; you may get it by cracking the nuts and putting the meat between hot tongs, and pressing it moderately over a small vessel. Put the oil on your lips at night—this has given considerable relief.

To cure the Toothache.

Take the powder of wild celendine root (called by some sullindine) and put it on and in the tooth a number of times, if it comes handy, and it will cure the toothache, or cause it to fall out in a few days. Hold the tea or juice of the herb

H

to the tooth, or you may chew the weed, and it will cure the toothache.

To cure Warts.

Rub on the juice of wild celendine frequently, and it will cure them.

To cure the Earache.

Black sheep's wool dipped in rum and put in the ear is good. Black negro's wool dipped in rum is much better. If you have not rum, dip it in strong vinegar. Sometimes a teaspoonful of rum has been put into the ear with good effect, and repeated time after time when the ear aches—this has given considerable relief.

For the Dysentery.

Take a bushel or more of cobs, and burn them to ashes, boil the ashes in water sufficiently, settle and strain off the lie, boil down 3 or 4 quarts to one, so that it may not freeze. Give a teaspoonful once an hour for a few times. This is likewise a remedy for worms. A few teaspoonfuls put into dough, is esteemed better than pearlash.

For the Dysentery, when powerfully seized.

Make a good tea of sumach berrys—give it once an hour, as occasion may require.

For the Dysentery.

Take two or three stalks of mairtail, simmer them in milk, enough for a potion.

For a person that is in a decline, & that has a cough.

Take a large onion, or in that proportion, slice them fine and cover them tight, boil them to a pap, then put in one pint of good milk and salt it a little, and scald in a little Indian meal—

take a pint of this when you go to bed, or as much as your stomach can bear—sleep on your back, if you can. By thus poulticing the bowels, deliverance has been wrought when medical skill has failed. Continue this till quite well.

Cure for Corns on the feet.

Chew a few white beans to a pap, then rub them on your corns smartly for five or six minutes—take some more thus chewed and bind them on the corns for a plaster, and thus do three or four times.

It has been said that spider's web wet in good vinegar and bound on the corns a few times, will cure them.

For the Wind Colick.

Take a table spoonful of dragon root, made fine and mixed with molasses, for a grown person, and for lesser persons in proportion, according to stature and complaint.

For the mother Colick—it is sometimes called Hysterick Colick.

Take a limb from the most pleasant sour apple tree, as big as your little finger, take the bark of this for six inches, put it into a teacup of boiling water, or a little more, setting it off the fire, stirring it while it comes the colour of weakish tea—take one teacup full and give it to the person, and it will produce fearful feelings, working a real cure.

For a breach in persons, or creatures.

Take the oil of hen's eggs, when it is first done, and oint the place once a day for two or three days. In order to get this oil, take four or six eggs, placing them in a spider or frying pan over a suitable fire, placing one edge of the vessel off the fire, and a little lower, pressing the eggs down, after a suitable time, with a flat piece of iron or earthen, till the oil runs out sufficiently, peradventure a spoonful or more.

To prevent Mortification.

Take a handful of hops, boil them strong, stirring in wheat or rye bran, sufficient for a poultice. This has cured when the physician's skill has failed. Repeat this poultice if necessary.

For the Billious or any other Colick.

Take the roots of milk weed, dry them without washing—pound them up fine and sift them—apply a table spoonful to a person. This has cured when the physician's skill failed.

For the Rheumatism.

Take four ounces of logwood, steep it in three pints of water till it becomes one, then add one quart of rum—take a glass three times a day.

For the Rheumatism.

Take one ounce of dry garget root, split it up fine and put it into a quart of new rum; when the strength is sufficiently out, let the patient take half a common glass full of the liquor at a time, three times a day, morning, noon and night. Repeating this quantity four or five times, has effected a cure in obstinate cases.

For the Rheumatism.

One quart of smart weed steeped in one quart of water, not let it come to a boil, then strain it clean—take one glass, and put half a glass of milk with it, and take it every morning for nine, and it is a sure antidote; or take the same quantity in one quart of spirits—take a glass at a time nine mornings.

For the Rheumatism.

Take one gill of neat's foot oil, and two gills of brandy—simmer these together, stirring it till they mix—then take it off the fire, put in one beef's gall and one glass of spirits of turpentine; bathe with it once or twice in a day, and take inwardly brandy made strong with mustard seed, say half a glass or more as they can bear.

Rheumatic Ointment.

Take a point of beef's gall, and half a pint of sweet oil, one ounce of camphor gum, half an ounce spirits turpentine—put them together in a bottle—set it in a warm oven—shake them together—oint the part affected.

For the Jaundice.

For the jaundice, white ash bark, off the north side roots, Indian roots and yellow roots, dry them, pound them to a powder, take three table spoonfuls of each sort, and put them into half a pint of molasses, then take one spoonful at a time three mornings, and miss three mornings, until you take it nine times.

For the Dysentery.

Take one large mullen leaf or two small ones, and simmer it in a tea cup of new milk till you get the strength out—apply it to the patient, repeating it two or three times if necessary.

For the Dysentery.

Take the juice of black cherries, either in rum or without—apply it sufficiently.

A tea made of low running briars, is said to be good for the dysentery.

For the Rheumatism.

Take the bones of an old horse, no matter if they have laid out twenty years—take them and pound them with an axe or hammer till you have got a sufficient mess, boil them in a kettle genttly and sufficiently—after cooling it till about blood warm, put your hand on the top of it a few times, and rub on what sticks to your hand.

Cure for the Yellow Jaundice.

You will take a large handful of horseredish root, a handful of prickly ash bark, a handful of black cherry tree bark, and a double handful of hops, and put them into two gallons of cider, (let the cider be cold) and let it steep twenty four hours. This you will find to be a certain cure for the yellow jaundice.

DAVID MUNGER.

It has cured when bordering on the black jaundice, and when troubled with the bloody urine. You will remember to take one gill once in three hours every day.

For Numbness.

Take tamarack, or bald spruce bark, and a quantity of ginseng root, and put them into one quart of Holland gin.

Another for Numbness.

Take sage, put it into good brandy and put it in a warm oven after baking.

For the Billious Complaint.

Take the bark of white ash roots, cut it fine and fill a quart mug with it, then boil it in water until it has got the strength from the bark—then take two thirds of a teacup full of the tea in the morning, and repeat the dose once an hour till it operates as a puke, and physic, which clears the bile from the stomach and bowels and leaves the body in health.

For a weak Stomach.

Take Indian root, take out the pith and slice it fine, put it in a kettle, and add molasses to it, one quart to a peck of the root, and boil it moderately until it is soft, then put it into a platter and sit it in an oven just warm enough to dry it, use it constantly for eating.

To prevent Mortification.

Take dogmacklemus leaves and ox balm, boil them and lay them on. This has cured when the skill of physicians has failed.

For Bursts.

Take bog onion, cumfrey, solomon's-seal, life of man, sarsaparilla, not-grass, shepherds spouts, (a large proportion of the bog onion,) boil them well together, strain it off and cool it. Add one pint of molasses to a gallon.

Dr Ford's Receipt for a Fever.

To break up a fever with cold water. First wash the patient all over with salt and water cold. When the fever is rising, apply a cloth doubled, wet in fresh cold water ten minutes; this do three times, washing the cloth clean and airing it, then apply a dry cloth thirty minutes. Thus continue the cloths till the fever abates. If the fever returns again, use the cloth as before mentioned. Apply a draught to the feet. Physick should be taken to keep the body in proper order.

A Receipt made of that wonderful root possessing many names. The names are,

Sweet root, Indian root, petty morrill, life of man, spikenard, cory come.

To prevent Mortification in brutes or human beings.

Make a tea of this root and wash frequently.

Receipt for a Weak Stomach.

Take the plumbs of this wonderful root, possessing many names, and put them in spirits, and make the spirits strong with them, take it from time to time. The effect will be good.

For weakness in men, or female weakness or weaknesses.

Take two or two and a half pails full of double tansy closely packed in a pot, put on a tin still, draw out two quarts of essence, add a quarter of spirits or less, so as to keep it, cork it up. Take a glass at a time, half an hour before eating, two or three times a day, & thus continue till you take a quart or more. If you use single tansy you must use twice the quantity above mentioned.

For Ague or Cold in the Face, or any part of the body.

Take the life of man root and pound it fine, and simmer it in new milk, stir in a little wheat flower so as to make it hold together. Apply it as a poultice.

Another for the Ague in the Face.

Take rum, mix it with wheat flower, lay it on for a poultice. This has performed great cures.

To dissolve the stone in the bladder.

Take golden rod tea, by simmering and not by boiling. When the tea is made simmer twelve honey bees in the tea for a man, nine for a woman.

Another for the stone in the bladder.

Make a tea of juniper berries and noble pine, called by some pip cisseway, by simmering it together without boiling, put gin with it; and take it sufficiently.

For the Gravel.

Take medicamentum, sometimes called Haarlem oil, you will get it in small bottles at the Apothecaries.

To cure the Itch.

Take pulverized black pepper, ginger an equal quantity, one gill in the gross, put one quarter of elecampane root, mix them with oil of turpentine, so that it is moist, put a piece as large as a bean in the palm of your hand, and rub them hard together, and smell of your hands as you would a pinch of snuff, for one week.

To cure a swelling caused by a broken joint.

Take wormwood, pound it up and wet it with rum or brandy, and put it on and wear it till it is dry. Take red clover and dragon root, and pound them together and spread them on a plaster; spread sour cream on the top of it and put it on. This has proved to be a cure.

For the Jaundice, when the person has got nigh the black Jaundice or Consumption.

For jaundice, take moose miss, beginning at the but and cut it into chips to the amount of four quarts, put it in an iron pot, boil it three hours, recruiting the water, leaving at last one quart of liquor, and throw the chips on the ground. You may drink this quart in a day if you are able; if you find it helps you, continue the same till you get quite well. For a cough or a cold, use it in the same manner.

For the Cancer.

Take red ash bark and burn it to ashes on a rock, then make lie and boil it to salts, and when the cancer is raw, pound the salts to powder and put a little into it, if there is proud flesh.

Make a salve of red clover heads, pick them when in full bloom, and boil them about three hours, then press them and strain the water, then boil it down gently. When about one pint, then put it into earthen, simmer it down gently and not burn it, then spread a plaster on a linen rag and apply it to the cancer.

Make a tea of clover heads, for constant drink, and drink nothing else, and wash the sore as often as you dress it in the same. Gather the clover heads when in full bloom, and dry them well without dew, if you have need to keep them.

Make an ointment of fresh butter, simmer the butter on a fire to an oil, then apply it to the sore, round the edge with a feather, once in two days, and oftener if it does not heal too fast.

Take garget berries when ripe, and squeeze the juice out, and put it into an earthen pot and set it in the sun, and dry it to a salve: then apply it to the cancer on a clean linen rag, if you can get them.

For a person that is in a Decline.

For any person that is in a decline and has a cough, and raises blood, buy a bottle of Riga balsam, and take five or six drops at a time, and keep gaining until you can take a teaspoonful at a time. Take white coharsh roots, Indian roots, and black alder berries, and make a strong bitter, and put them into new rum, equal in quantity and sweeten it with molasses, and take it morning & evening, or at eleven o'clock. Take all the above mentioned balsam before you meddle with the bitter. Take it in the morning.

One quart of sweet oil taken by a child before they are ten years old is said to cure the phthisic.

Gold thread tea sweetened with honey is good for the Canker; drink a little and soak or swab the mouth.

Fill a barrel with green mullen leaves, then with new cider, drink it out for the phthisic or asthma, after it is worked.

For the Rheumatism.

Coak-ash root, a sovereign cure for the rheumatism. Take a handful of the roots, put them into one quart of brandy, and let them stand until well steeped, say 48 hours; then wash the part affected with the brandy by the fire, and drink of the brandy inwardly, say half a glass or less as the person can bear, and apply red baize to the part where the pain is seated, and follow this if you wish to be cured of the rheumatism. Do it night and morning.

Make a tea of the same root, and it will cure the colick, or any pain in the bowels or stomach.

For the rheumatism, when settled in the joints, take cedar boughs, boil them in brandy till the bark comes off, take out the twigs and boil it down to a salve, then spread a plaster & apply it.

For the Rheumatism.

Take a handful of rusty iron, put it into strong vinegar, and let it set a sufficient space of time; then rub the pained part every night when you are in bed, or going to bed.

Cough.

Take one egg, put in good vinegar sufficient to cover it, let it set while the vinegar eats the egg, take the skin out, and it is fit for use; set it up, sweeten it with honey or loaf sugar, and take one spoonful at a time.

Humours.

For Humours, take meadow fern, it is sometimes called bay-bush, make a tea of the twigs and leaves, as strong as you would common tea; and stronger if needed. Drink it with your victuals continually, as you would tea, or at any time in the course of the day. It is said to be a sovereign remedy for humours.

This bush generally grows round water, and one kind of it may be known by its golden bur or bud when it is grown; either kind will answer.

Jaundice.

For the Jaundice, take lime not slacked, soak it in spring water, drink a glass in the morning and at 11 o'clock.

A. Brown's receipt for the Dysentery.

Take one new laid egg, loaf sugar the size of the egg, one teaspoon full of gumarabic, pulverized fine, and half a glass of brandy or Holland gin, mix them well together. The above to be taken at one dose by persons full grown, six times a day; and for a child accordingly. If the patient be thirsty, drink freely of balm tea.

Cough.

For a cough, take one spoon full of dragon root, one spoonful of flax seed, one of the top of new milk, and one of honey; each a teaspoonful of these mixed.

For the aforementioned Cough, take one teaspoonful once in an hour, if the cough is hard, if not, take it in two or three hours.

Another for Cough.

Take onions, cut them fine and boil them to a pap, put in two or three garlics, if you have them, strain them through a fine cloth, sweeten it with honey or loaf sugar, put gin sufficient to preserve it, and bottle it up. Take a small quantity at night when you go to bed.

For a Cough, yellow dock root and burdock root steeped in new rum as usual: take half a glass of the bitter in the morning and at 11 o'clock. Make a tea of clover heads, and take it frequently.

Gravel.

For the Gravel, take one pound of honey and a quart of spring water that runs to the north, put them into a kettle, set it over the fire, stir it and skim it till it boils, then cool it, do so three times, then give one glass at a time three times in a day, if needed.

For the Gravel, take bald spruce balls and make a strong tea, and drink once an hour, and it will relieve the distress.

Toothache.

For the toothache, take moose-wood bark, boil it, and hold it in the mouth, and it will kill the marrow of the tooth.

For the tooth-ache, take onions, or an onion, roast it soft, put as much salt as onion, make a poultice and bind them on the wrists.

Piles.

For the Piles, mullen tops in bloom; make a tea of it in water, wet a rag in the same, grate some hemlock turpentine that gathers on the cracked part of the tree, on the rag for a plaster; apply the same.

Weakness.

For inward weakness and female complaints, take one ounce of white corhash roots, dry them, and pound them to powder, and put them into two quarts of new rum and half a pint of molasses—shake them together and let it stand twenty-four hours, then take half a wine glass full at a time two or three times a day, and if exposed to cold, at other times also.

Hungry Evil.

For the evil, take garden wormwood, hemlock boughs, peppermint herbs, elder flowers, penny-royal herbs, put them in water, and draw the tea out of them; this is the medicine for steaming the face when a person has a cold or swelling under the chops.

Tobacco simmered in hog's fat, rubbed on for the cancer or humour in the breast.

Catarrh.

For the catarrh, make and take snuff from the bark of bayberry root.

Cracked and Swelled Hands.

Red pitch-pine gum is good for cracked fingers.
Fresh pitch-pine turpentine, applied to a swelling is good.

Asthma.

Take the lights of a fox, wash them clean and dry them, then grind them to a powder, put them with two quarts of good brandy, let the whole stand twenty-four hours, then

I

begin to take it, one wine glass full in the morning on an empty stomach, and so continue.

Piles.

The symptoms of a disease inclining to piles, itching in the hollow of the hands and feet, and from that to a prickling in the mouth, lips, swelling, &c. a shortness of breath, faintness, and fainting, if not prevented will turn to fits.

A real Cure.

Spring water from the north side of a hill, take one gallon of this water, and put it in a tea-kettle, then fill it up with angelico and rue, then stop up the tea-kettle and boil it down to two quarts, then take out the herbs, and put in one pound of brown sugar, then let it come to a scald, then set it by till blood warm, then put in rum enough to preserve it, then put it in bottles and put it down cellar, be sure to put the stopple in loose, then drink one glass of it at a time three times in a day, repeating this till you get well.

Pains in the Stomach and Bowels.

Tansy and horsemint rubbed to a powder, mixed with molasses, for a cramp or pain in the stomach.

Mustard seed and molasses, for a pain in the bowels.

Scalds.

For a scald, take smart beer emptings, warm it blood warm, and thicken it with Indian meal sufficient for a poultice, and let it be applied every half hour until the fire is drawn out, which if immediately applied, the third or fourth commonly gives relief unless very bad, and then it must be continued longer. N. B. Apply a little oil to prevent the poultice sticking.

Burns and Freezes.

For burns and freezes, take white oak bark one half a pot full, then white pine bark about one quarter as much as of the oak, sassafras sprouts a small handful; fill the pot full of water, boil the water away to one half, take out the barks and sprouts, then boil the water about three quarters away, then it is fit for use to wash the frozen or burnt parts.

Worms.

For worms, double tansy—the juice of it green, mixed with rum and molasses, or distilled spirits of the tansy taken on sugar.

For worms, take poplar bark pounded fine, mixed with molasses.

To cure the sick or nervous Head-Ache.

Take one ounce of the rind of white pine bark; one ounce of the rind of hemlock bark; one ounce of baberry bark, off the root; one half ounce of sassafras bark, off the root; and one half ounce of black cherry tree bark, grind these to a powder, put them into two quarts of good French brandy, shake them up three days and take one table spoonful in the morning and at 11 o'clock.

Sore Eyes.

For sore eyes—When the eyes are very much inflamed with heat, it is necessary to cool the inflammation. Cure—Take one pint of barley, and boil it until it cracks open; then take out the barley and pound it in a mortar as fine as you can while it is warm, then boil it again with some English turnip, sliced fine; when it is boiled very soft, take the barley and turnips together and strain them through a thin cloth, the same as you would hog's fat, then take a linen cloth and wet it in the stuff thus strained, fold it up three or four times, and bind the cloth thus wet on the eyes at night when you go to bed, and repeat it as often as you find it necessary.

The poultice above described is an eminent medicine to cure the broken breast, to ease the pain, and subdue the inflammation.

Indigestion.

For any person whose food lies hard, or does not digest, take pigeon's or partridge's gizzards, the inside skin, (pigeon's is much the best,) and dry them and pound them to a powder, and take a tea spoonful at a time, and it will answer a good purpose in a relaxed state.

Dysentery.

For the dysentery, take spleen roots and put them into clear cold water, steep it strong, and not let it come to a boil; apply to a patient, one table spoonful if a grown person, and a child of ten years a tea spoonful once in half an hour.

Tansy, horsemint, and fever bush, made into a tea sweetened with molasses, is good for the dysentery.

Cold in the Breast.

For a cold in the breast, take mutton tallow, beeswax and saffron; simmer these together in equal proportions, put to it one spoonful of rum, make it into a plaster, put it on the pap.

Colick.

For the wind cholic, take a large puff ball, or two or three small ones, put them into one pint of skimmed milk, and boil them about half an hour; apply one half of it to the patient at a time.

Cancer.

For a Cancer, take garget root, make a tea of it and drink of it, and wash the Cancer in the same; grate the root on a wet rag for a plaster. When the leaves of the garget grow (if needed) make a salve of the leaves by putting them between pewter, and setting it in the sun, carrying it in at night. Continue thus till it is sufficiently turned.

Rheumatism.

For the Rheumatism, use a tea of garget root, stronger and stronger, till it physicks you—after a pause, repeat it if needed.

Jaundice.

For the Jaundice, take some soot off the chimney, (stone soot is much the best) where it is glossed so as to shine; simmer it in water, & take a sufficient quantity.

Felon.

To cure a felon, take soot and salt, the yolk of an egg; an equal proportion of these; make them into a poultice, put it on four times a day, for four days running, if needed.

For a second poultice, to cleanse the sore; take honey, the yolk of an egg, and wheat flour.

For a salve, take cream, simmer houseleek and camomile therein, and green of elder, and a little beeswax.

Another for a Felon.

Take dragoon root, make it fine in vinegar for a poultice, either grating or slicing and simmering it.

Houseleek is good to take fire out of burns, to prevent blistering, and will cure the corns, by applying the juice or mashing it, and binding it up a few times.

Dog and Serpent Bite.

For the bite of a mad dog or serpent, or sting of a serpent, take the yolk of an egg, and the same quantity of honey mixed together, grated over with dragoon root, mix it up together with flour sufficient for a poultice—apply it two or three times to the bite or stinged place.

For the bite of a serpent, take blue flag root and pound it well, and wet it with chamber lie, and apply a poultice three times, or as often as it dries.

Bite on Creatures.

For mad dog bite on creatures, take scull cap and lobelia, make them into a tea, and give it sufficiently to the creature.

Fever or Cold.

For a fever, or a sudden cold, take one gill of wild valerian roots, put them into half a pint of cold water, simmer it on the fire and not let it boil, then apply it to the patient, one gill at a time, if a strong natured person more, and give it once an hour for three hours, and it will break a fever commonly.

For a Mare that has nots, or curdles in her bag, or for a Cow in the same condition.

Take blacksmith's cinder from his forge, no matter if it has laid out for a number of years; pound it up fine and boil it in water one hour. Bathe the bag with this water as hot as you can put it on with your hand for ten or fifteen minutes, twice a day. This is superior to other things used. It is good for a wound in a Cow's bag, bathed in the same manner: and it is also good for the garget in the cow's bag.—This will cure in four of five days; if not, garget the cow with a piece of dry garget root in the following manner: Thrust up your penknife between the thick skin of the lowest part of the dulap, an inch and a half for a middling creature; then prepare a piece of garget an inch & a half long, tie a string to the lower end of it, sharp the upper end, and thrust it in the place you have made, half an inch above the lower part of the hole, and let the string hang out. Green garget will have no effect.

For a Fever Sore, or any old Scrofulous Sore.

Take the water out of a Blacksmith's trough, where he quenches his iron, and warm the water by quenching hot iron in it as warm as you can bear it, and bathe your sores with it for two months. This generally cures in this time, and sometimes much sooner.

A very extraordinary receipt for a Broken Bone, Bruised Joint, Sprain, or any bruise on persons or creatures.

For a broken bone, take beef brine and Roman wormwood, boil them half an hour and bathe it on the man's wound, twice a day sufficiently. This has healed to the astonishment of the physician. If the pain is great, do it more frequently.

For the Sprain of an Ox or Horse, or for a Bruise, or Bruised Joint.

Make a tea of bitter sweet vine, or root; simmer it in a little hog's fat, and wash the bruised part frequently. This is said to be very good. Bathe it twice a day, hot.

For Mad Dog Bite.

Take alismusplantago. This grows in the edges of lakes, rivers ponds or brooks; It puts up one stock above one foot high, then it presents one leaf, sending up by the side of that a spindle that blows out with blue blossoms in July.

The root has a small bunch in the middle from whence proceeds many small roots. Dig this up, dry it, make it fine and sprinkle a potion of it on a piece of bread and butter. This cures man or beast, the second or third time given.

To break a Sore.

When you wish to break a sore by poulticing, take scavice leaves and viney malace that grows about the door, half and half of these, jam or cut them fine and simmer them in water until tender, then stir in Indian meal for a poultice, repeat this poultice as often as necessary. It is said to be very good.

For the Itch or Salt Rheum, or any Humour.

Take half a pint of the spirits of turpentine, a pound of fresh butter, and a quarter of a pound of Burgundy pitch, for the summer, two ounces for winter. Take half an ounce of mutton tallow, and as much bees wax. Put these in a small vessel, and simmer them for three hours moderately, stirring it continually; when done and cooling, put in one ounce of red precipitate ground fine, stirring it moderately till cold. If you burn it, it is spoiled.

Rub on this ointment when going to bed, on places where you itch or break out. A week for the salt Rheum generally cures, sometimes it takes longer.

To cure vegetable Poison.

Take wild celendine and jam it up, and rub it on frequently; this is said to give great relief. Some have called it snap weed. Some have used white scabish in the same manner.

A tea made of sweet fern and wash frequently has sometimes cured—and meadow firn used in the same manner has sometimes cured. You may drink the tea of either of the ferns safely. Also, good strong soap suds made with good spring water and bathed on ten or fifteen minutes as hot as you can bear it for five or six nights generally cures.

When vegetable poison is first taken, bathe with rum, or put a quarter of a pound of sulphur into a junk bottle, and fill it with rum; cork it tight, put it into a pot and boil it a considerable time. Bathing with this when first taken prevents its operation—this gives very good relief after it blisters and becomes sore.—A poultice made of wheat flour, put on the feet, has given some relief.

BAITING.

BEE BAIT.

For bee bait—take the oil of fennel and amber, and oil of rhodiam; an equal proportion of these and put about two drops to a pound of strained honey, and boil about one gill of chamber lie, and put it in with it; put into the box grudgeons of comb and two or three pieces of comb. The oil of white oak acorn is supposed to be superior, put in an equal proportion with the others, if you can get it.

This is an English art of hunting the bee, and is superior to our common way; for the bee will be fond of this box; whereas he would desert the other box, prepared in the common manner, and go to the flowers. When you line the bee, wait till he comes back three or four times then he will go straight from the box.

FISH BAIT.

For catching fish—one half ounce the oil of fennel to four drops of the oil of rhodiam, and about twenty drops of the oil of amber, and mix them together in a bottle and cork it tight, and drop a small drop on or into the bait.

This is an English art of fishing, and has caused the fish to bite at the hook thus fixed, when they would not meddle with any other in the company.

FOX BAIT.

For fox bait—the oil of amber, one ounce, and ten or fifteen drops of the oil of rhodiam—mix them together, and apply it to the trap and bed, or on a stump or stake.

Make the bed of sifted chaff, about the bigness of a riddling seive or hogshead head; do not spit nor make water about your bed, nor step all about it. Blot out some of your tracks if necessary—put two or three pieces of old iron into your bed when you first make it, and the fox will not be afraid.

The pieces that you put on your bed should be fine; toasted cheese and toasted liver is good, and the insides of fowls and creatures is sometimes used. The liver of swine toasted, is the best kind of bait for them; if you rub this toasted on the bottom of your shoes, when you go to the bed, the fox will follow the track to the bed. Nuxvomity, melted or otherwise, put on to the bottom of your shoes will produce the same effect. Melt a good portion of this nuxvomity, if you see fit to poison them to death, and dip some large pieces of bait in it, and they will eat it and will seldom get more than forty rods when they will die—but if you please to take them as above directed, clean your trap of all rust or blood and smoke it thoroughly by putting a handful of hog's scraps on a shovel of coals, and hold the trap over the smoke, and be careful when you sit it or carry it to the bed not to get the smoke off. This is preferable to any other way of fixing the trap.

PIGEON BAIT.

Pigeon bait—Sassafras tree bark off the root, and buds and berries—boil them well and soak the wheat in the water, to draw the pigeons.

The oil of white oak acorn is supposed to be superior to any thing, if a right use be made thereof, to draw them until winter.

For pigeon bait, one half an ounce of the oil of fennel, four drops of the oil rhodiam, and about fifteen drops of anise oil, and about thirty drops of the spirits of nitre; mix them together and take a pint of West-India rum, one half pint of molasses, and a spoonful of honey—shake them together, and keep them corked in a bottle. Put into two quarts of wheat one table spoonful in your common baitings.

Take one tea spoonful anise seed, one tea spoonful of cumin seed, one tea spoonful of phynegreg seed, and pound them to powder, and one table spoonful fine salt, one table spoonful of India sugar, and put them into two quarts of wheat, shut in a box and let it stand over night, then give in the afternoon before catching.

When you make your bed to bate pigeons, make it level and smooth, do not spit about it, nor make water about it, do not handle guns nor powder about it.—When you catch your pigeons be careful to put away all blood and feathers, and cover them up.

EXPLANATION OF WORDS.

Pennyroyal Water—Is gotten from the herb by distillation.

Lung Wort—Is found on the north side of white oak and maple trees; it best on the oak. A tea made of it and taken at night, delivers from a cold.

Hurds—Means tow, or old ropes picked to pieces to stop up the horses foot with.

To a Suppuration—Means to a head, or fit to open. "*Emollient*" means softening.

A Seton in the most depending part—Means rowel in the lowest part.

Intestines—The bowels.

Nitre—Is salt Petre.

Bay Salt—is made out of the water of the ocean by boiling down.

Bay Leaves—probably means the leaves of the bay bush, called by some meadow Ferne.

Concocted together—Means boiled together.

Alkaline Substances—Is potash, pearlash, or lie.

Sallad Oil—Is Olive oil.

London Treacle—is composed of five or six different articles or more, and sold at the Apothecaries.

Venetian soap—Is Castile soap made in Venice, & sold by the Apothecaries.

Take 1 pound of Blood from the Jugular vein which is a pint. The Jugular is the neck vein.

Licorice Ball—Is made of Licorice root boiled down in water with good molssses, strained and boiled down to a candy or substance for a ball.

Yellow Basilicon—Is made of the following articles: Hog's lard, eight parts, Rosin, five parts, Bees wax, two parts, simmered together and strained.

The bite of a green or yellow spider is fatal unless the juice of plantain is seasonably applied.

The Indians cure the Dysentery with sassafras in the most obstinate cases.

CONTENTS.

FIRST PART.—OF HORSES.

	Page		Page
Broken wind,	18	Hoof-bound,	25
Bots,	18	Health,	6
Bleeding,	19	Lampers,	4
Clysters,	13	Nicking,	6
Colts,	4	Pricked Hoofs,	20
Cramp,	13	Ring-bone,	22
Clap in the back Sinews,	17	Remarks on Travelling,	26
Choosing a Horse,	25	Seed Horses,	4
Docking,	5	Stabling,	9
Eyes Sore,	23	Staggers,	11
Exercise,	8	Strangury,	12
Food,	7	Shoulder Strain,	16
Frenzy,	11	Scouring,	19
Fever,	12	Sore Back,	19
Fistula,	14	Spavins,	21
Filing teeth,	23	Splents,	21
Glanders,	10	Scratches,	23
Gripes,	18	Strains in the Hip,	24
Gravelled Hoofs,	20	Stifle,	24
Hide bound,	17	Worms,	18
Horse Ointment,	21	Wind-galls,	22
Horse Ail,	10	Yellows,	12
Hip-shot,	24		

SECOND PART.—OF CATTLE.

	Page		Page
Bladders,	30	Murrian,	29
Blains,	31	Overflowing of the Gall,	32
Barbs,	32	Overheat,	36
Broken Horns,	33	Poisons,	31
Broken Legs,	33	Pissing Blood,	30
Bleeding,	36	Scab,	30
Cough,	29	Scurf,	30
Cud lost,	33	Teeth Loose,	32
Calving,	35	Taping,	34
Cows' Bags,	35	Taint,	30
Calves that Scour,	35	Tail Sick,	36
Falling of the Matrice,	34	Vomiting,	32
Fever,	28	Wind Colick,	29
Garget,	30	Worms,	31
Horn ail,	31	Wens,	33

THIRD PART.—OF SHEEP.

	Page		Page
Cud Lost,	38	Plague,	37
Cough,	39	Poison,	38
Fever,	38	To Preserve from Rot,	39
Milk to Increase,	38	Scab Rot,	38
Maggots, to kill,	38	Staggers,	39

FOURTH PART.—OF SWINE.

	Page		Page
Catarrh,	40	Issues,	41
Drenches,	40	Measles,	40
Fever,	40	Swine Pox,	40

ADDITIONS.

	Page
To cure a Horse of the Bots,	42, 53, 54, 58, 59
A cure for the Horn-ail in Cattle,	43
To cure a horse of the Heaves,	43, 47, 59
A cure for Cows and Oxen troubled with the garget,	44
For a creature choaked,	45
Cure for a Castrated Horse, sore necked Ox, or galled Horse,	45
For a foundered Horse by eating grain,	45
For a Horse foundered by drinking Water,	45
For scouring of Cattle or Horses,	46
For the overflow of the gall,	46
For the Glands,	46
For a Bone Spavin,	47
Cure for Horses of the Pool-evil and Thistalow,	47
To cure the Spavin,	47
To cure the scowers in Cattle and Horses,	48
To cure the Ring-Bone,	48, 53
For Ring Bones and hard Spavins,	48
For soft Spavins,	48
For a galled Horse,	48
Proper conduct with Mares,	49
To make the most valuable green Ointment	51
To make the valuable Copperas water, to wash or syringe, or drench sores on Horses,	52
For a stoppage or Dry Belly Ache in a Horse or Ox,	52, 54
A cure for Ring Bones,	53
A cure for Wind Spavins, or Blood Spavins,	53
For the Murrian in Cattle,	54
For a stoppage in the Manifold of a neat creature	54
The symptoms of the Water Garget,	55
The symptoms of the Yellow Garget,	55
For the Castration of Horses,	55
For the Staggers in Horses,	56
To cure Oxen poisoned by eating Kill Lamb,	56
To cure a Horse of the Canker,	56
For the Gripes,	57
To stop a horse from Bleeding at the nose or elsewhere,	57
To cure the Barbs in Horses,	57
A description of Savine and Cedar,	59
For the Castration of any creature,	60
To cause a Horse to vomit,	60
To keep flies from tormenting a Horse,	61
The disease in the Horse called the flying Worm, Tetter, or Ring Worm.	61
For a Horse Gravelled,	62
To cure a Horse of the Flux or Scowers,	62
Treatment of Horses, &c.	62

MEDICAL RECEIPTS.

For a child that is stuffed up,	65
For Corns on the feet,	65, 67, 80, 82, 87
To cure the Asthma,	65, 70
For the Cramp Rheumatism,	66

	Page
For the Ague in the Face,	66, 92
For the Wind Colick,	66, 87
For the Dysentery,	66, 67, 74, 78, 81, 82, 83, 86, 89, 96, 99
For the Dysentery when powerfully seized,	86
A receipt for that disease which is properly called a Stoppage in the water.	66
To prevent Fits,	67
To take a Film off the Eye,	67
For Sore Eyes,	68, 73, 74, 99
Symptoms of the Maw worm,	68
A Plaster for a pain in the back or side,	69
For a pain in the Stomach, or for the Billious Colick, or for any other Colick, and for the wind in the Stomach,	69, 100
For the Jaundice complaint in persons, and for the overflow of the gall in creatures,	69
To cure the Sore Throat,	70
Cure for Fever and Ague,	70, 83, 101
For the King's Evil,	70
A good and wholesome physick for those that need,	71
To cure hard drinking,	76
For the Asthma and Cough—this is a cure even if it has been of long standing,	72
For an inflamed, feverish, swelled leg,	72
To kill Worms in Children,	72
For Worms,	73, 84
For Consumptive complaints,	73
For a humour in the leg by a hurt or strain,	73
For the Ague Fever,	74
For an inward Fever,	74
Cure for a Cold,	74, 78
Cure for Consumption,	75
Worm Pills,	75
Cure for puking up food,	75
Cure for a bad Cough,	75, 78, 80, 83, 95, 96
To make a Plaster to be put on the bottom of the feet, when the head is pressed with hypocondriack and humour,	75
To cure the Toothache,	76, 85
For children when they have worms and the Worm Fever,	76
For the Rheumatism in the Cords, Muscles or Joints,	76
A sovereign remedy for the Jaundice,	76, 100
For the Catarrh,	77, 97
For the Piles,	77, 97, 98
For the Cancer or Scrofula humour,	77, 93, 100
For inward humour or Rheumatism,	77
To heal an old sore,	77
For the Canker,	78, 81, 83
For a Fever,	78, 80
For a green Wound or Cut,	78
For the Dropsy,	78, 82
To kill Ringworms,	79
Dr. John Smith's receipt for curing the Toothache,	79
Mr. Daniel Tenney's receipt to cure Sore Eyes,	79
To cure a Felon or Whitlow before it is ulcerated,	80, 100
For a weak Stomach and Consumptive complaints,	80

	Page
The best Plaster for weakness or pain in the back,	80
For the Relax and Dysentery—by James Scammon,	81
For Burns, to prevent blistering,	82, 98
For the Rheumatism,	82, 83, 88, 89, 90, 95, 100
For a Cut, to prevent soreness,	82
For Deafness,	84
Cure for Worms, or any person whose victuals hurt them,	84
To cure a Felon after it is ulcerated,	84
To cure a Whitlow or Burn,	85
Dr. Morse's receipt to draw a Felon to a head,	85
To harden or help your fingers when they are cracked by drawing a thread through them,	85
For cracked or sore Lips,	85
To cure Warts,	86
For a person that is in a decline, and that has a Cough,	86
For the Mother Colick—it is sometimes called Hysterick Colick,	87
For a breach in persons or creatures,	87
To prevent Mortification,	88, 91, 92
For the Billious or any other Colick,	88
Rheumatick Ointment,	89
For the Jaundice,	89, 96
Cure for the Yellow Jaundice,	90
For Numbness,	90
For the Billious complaint,	90
For a weak Stomach,	91, 92
For Bursts,	91
Dr. Ford's receipt for a Fever,	91
For weakness in men, or female weakness or weaknesses,	92
For Ague or Cold in the face, or any part of the body,	92
To dissolve the Stone in the Bladder,	92
For the Gravel,	93, 96
To cure the Itch,	93, 102
To cure a swelling caused by a broken joint,	93
For the Jaundice when a person has got nigh the Black Jaundice or Consumption,	93
For the Cancer,	93
For a person in a decline,	94
Indigestion,	99
Humours,	96
Female Weakness,	97
Hungry Evil,	97
Cracked and Swelled Hands,	97
Pains in the Stomach and Bowels,	98
Scalds,	98
Dog and Serpent bite,	101
Bite on creatures,	101
For a Mare that has nots, or curdles in her bag,	101
For a Fever Sore, or any old Scrofulous Sore,	101
For Broken Bones, Bruised Joints, &c.	102
For the Sprain of an Ox or Horse,	102
For Mad Dog bite,	102
To break a Sore,	102
To cure vegetable poison,	102
For Baiting,	103

The following Receipts were received after the foregoing part of the book was printed.

A Receipt to cure Ring-bones in Horses.

Take toads and split them open, lay them all round the ankle or ankles where the ring bones are, swarth them on with a wide bandage and bind it with strong twine, fastening the ends sufficiently, then turn the horse out till he gets well.

This will take the hair off his ankles, but it will be likely to grow again.

There is a weed called *Slink weed,* by which the farmer has lost all his Calves and Colts, it being mixed with his grass or hay. This weed looks a little like lovage, and grows in wet places. Savin produces the same effect.

Mares, after foaling sometimes have knots or curdles in their bags.

Cure. Milk out as much of the milk as you can, and boil the leaves of lavender or spike therein, and wash her bag frequently with it warm; continue it every day until well. Let her drink be white water.

Also, previous to the horses' coming together, as mentioned in the 49th page, 10th line, let their drink be white water : and at night, after she has taken the horse, begin and continue her drink as above mentioned.

White water is supposed to be good clean soft running water, that will wash well which is supposed to be what Jewett calls fair water.

To Cure a Horse of a fresh Sore or Wound.

Take one quart of chamberlie, one spoonful of salt and three spoonsfull of good common soap, simmer these together sufficiciently and wash the

K

sore with it once a day; make a strong tea of white oak bark and wash with this once a day. You may wash with these different ingredients oftener than once a day if you see fit. Sweep soot out of the chimney and throw this all over the sore frequently, and wash it off when you wash the sore, this will prevent the proud flesh from growing.

This process has been known to heal the worst of wounds, and that speedily; if there is any hollow place in the sore that cannot be washed, drench it with a little piece of pork tied on the end of a stick dipped in the wash.

For the St. Anthony's Fire.

Take may weed or peppermint tea frequently after going to bed, steeped strong, and sweat six hours freely, then keep in a moderate sweat for five days, giving the peppermint or mayweed tea. Give the patient any thing to eat or to drink that he has an inclination for. This is as sure a remedy as any that I know of. When you come out of the sweat be careful not to take cold.

To stop a Felon, before it becomes ulcerated.

Take Scavis Leaves and simmer them in hogs fat, and put it on two or three times a day. This will cure it.

For a person that has bruised his flesh black and blue, or for a new bruise, or if the flesh be jamed open or cut open.

Pour on cold water out of a coffee pot or picher or any thing handy rubbing the wounded part with your hand all about, while you pour, as hard as you are able to bear it. Pour on five or six quarts twice a day if you are able to bear it, and thus continue till well. Wrap it up in a warm woollen cloth after bathing. This cures in a short time.

A strong tea of white oak bark bathed on a

black and blue wound, as hot as you can bear it when you begin, and bathe till the tea is cold. This has given immediate relief.

To cure Vegetable Poison.

Rub on a little of the spirits of turpentine two or three times and it will cure. Do not rub on but little for fear of weakening the joints.

The common practice of our modern Doctors.

A person is sick and sends for a doctor; the doctor comes and feels the pulse, inquires the complaints then tells them they are threatened with a fever, and he will try to throw it off, then gives a puke, takes his hat and goes away—next morning returns, tells them the fever is settled—it will run ten or fifteen days then deals out medicine, first Calomel and Rheubarb to be given, then takes camphor, magnesia, salt petre, what the point of a penknife will hold of each put together. This to be given every hour for five hours; then they give rheubarb and calomel; If the patient should be full of pain, or have pain at any time, they generally give opium in a fine powder or paregoric dops, which is opium and rum. Thus they continue in that way till the patient lives or dies.

To cure the Fever.

Give the patient two thirds of a tea cup full of good lobelia tea for a puke, and repeat it once every half hour till the stomach is cleared, put the patient to bed and sweat him well one day by giving peppermint, or mayweed, or pennyroyal tea. Either of these teas will do. After the first day's sweating, sweat moderately till the fever leaves them. Be careful not to take cold. This releaves from the canker in the mouth and bowels. Let the patient eat what he craves.

To make plasters for the Rheumatism.

Take the balsam of Hemlock, from the cracked or bruised part of the tree, mixed with the oil of hen's eggs, for a plaister.

Another plaster for the Rheumatism.

Take hemlock bows and white pine bows, in equal proportions—boil them till the balsam is off; then skim off the balsam, and boil it down thick enough to spread in a plaster.

For a weak Stomach.

Take the balsam of a tamarac tree. You will find it by whittling the wood open round the bruised part—take it on sugar or in molasses.

For the Dysentery.

Take a cork and burn it on coals, draw the tea out of this, and take it—it has wrought a cure when the skill of doctors has failed.

Cure for sore Eyes.

Take white vitriol as big as a white bean, the same quantity of loaf sugar, and a boiled or roasted egg; take out the yolk; put the vitriol and sugar into the white of the egg, and press them till the juice is all out—apply it to the eyes at night.

Cure for Poisoned Sheep and Cattle.

Raw eggs, says the American Farmer, given to sheep or cattle poisoned by eating laurel or ivy will effect a speedy cure. The dose for a sheep is one egg, for a cow four. When used for this purpose the shell of the egg is broken, and the yolk with as much of the white as is practicable is slipped down the animal's throat.

For the Horn Ail in Cattle.

Take of running Ivy, by some called Mercury, half a pound of vines and roots;—This is the thing that poisons men when they are mowing—Put it into a pail and a half of water, and boil it two thirds away, or in the same proportion for a greater or lesser quantity. Do not stand over the pot whilst it is boiling. Give the beast 3 or 4 junk bottles full at once according to the strength of the creature, and the cure is effected. This same medicine will also cure the Garget, and is good to give creatures in the spring to prevent diseases. half a pint or more of this tea given to a sheep a few times, that lingered and refused her meat before and after lambing, has been known to cure.

DR. JOHN WILLIAMS'
LAST LEGACY,
AND USEFUL
FAMILY GUIDE.

NEW-YORK:

1827.

PREFACE.

THE author of this little book has a desire to leave something for the good of his fellow creatures, and being sensible of soon retiring from time, and seeing no other opportunity to benefit the rising generation, hopes it will be kindly received—being a true and faithful statement of each Medicine and Cure.—It has been carefully minuted according to his own knowledge, and not from hearsay. He has endeavoured to state the true nature and virtue of each vegetable; and they may be used with the greatest safety and advantage.

JOHN WILLIAMS.

HERBAL.

1. *For the King's Evil.*

The King's Evil may be cured by a plant called the King's Evil weed. It grows in wild shady land, under almost all kinds of timber, and in the form of a plantain, but the leaves are smaller, and are spotted green and white—a very beautiful plant. When it goes to seed, there comes up one stalk in the middle of the plant, six or eight inches high, and bears the seed on the top of the stalk in a small round bud.

Take this, root and branch, pound it soft, apply it to the tumour for a poultice or salve, and let the patient drink a tea made of the same for constant drink. If the tumour is broken open, simmer the root and leaf in sweet oil and mutton tallow; strain it of, and add to it beeswax and rosin until hard enough for salve.—Wash the sore with liquor made of the herb, boiled, and apply the salve, and it will not fail a cure.

2. *The best remedy for the rattles in children.*

Take blood root, powder it, give the patient a small tea-spoonful at a dose; if the first does not break the bladder in half an hour, repeat again three times. This has not been known to fail curing.

3. *A valuable remedy for the Bilious Colic.*

Take of West India rum, one gill, of West India molasses, one gill, of hog's lard, one gill, and the urine of beast one gill; simmer well together. This composition will seldom fail of performing an effectual cure for life.

4. *For a Felon.*

Flue flag root and wild turnip root, a handful of each, stewed in half a pint of hog's lard—strain it off—add to it four spoonfuls of tar, and simmer them together. Apply this ointment to the felon till it breaks. Add beeswax and rosin to the ointment for a salve to dress it with after it is broken. This is an infallible cure, without losing a joint.

ADVERTISEMENT.

THE Author of this work is a native of New-York, and now resides in Washington county, in the easterly part of the state; he has for the most part of his life been engaged in the deepest study for restoring the health, and preserving the lives of his fellow creatures. For the attainment of this object he has travelled. To this end he has laboured, and for years has applied himself in the wilds of America, among the natives of the forest, where he has undergone all the horrors and deprivations incident to savage life, in order to collect and bring together that knowledge which should be instrumental in saving the lives and preserving the health of his fellow creatures.

Whilst among the Indians, the author was a particular inmate and confident of a native Indian, who had been instructed in all the arts of civilized life, and had the advantages of a liberal education, being a regular bred physician, in the medical department of the Pennsylvania university, established at Philadelphia, at once the most flourishing and respectable institution of the kind in the United States, and hardly excelled by any in Europe.—While with this Indian, the author of this work had not only an opportunity of learning the Indian method of treating disorders, and the medical virtues of the vegetable kingdom, but likewise of gaining much literary and scientific knowledge.

It is as clear as the sun at noon day, (and must be seen by all observers) that nature has provided in her minerals, animals and vegetables, an effectual remedy, if administered in season, for all the disorders incident to the human system. Of the two latter, the author has treated more particularly in his work, omitting mineral substances generally, on account of their poisonous quality—and which he thinks in a great measure ought to be laid aside. Should any recipe in the preceding pages answer the benevolent design of the writer—that of easing pain, curing diseases and prolonging life—the person so benefitted will be more than compensated for the price asked for this.

☞More than 8000 copies of this work have been sold within the last four months.

5. *For the Salt Rheum.*

Take swamp sassafras bark, boil it in water very strong, take some of the water and wash the part affected; to the remainder of the water add hog's lard, simmer it over a moderate fire till the water is gone. Oint the part affected after washing, (continued four days,) never fails of a cure.

6. *Salve for a Burn.*

Take wild lavender, the green of elder bark, cammomile, and parsley, and stew them in fresh butter, strain off, and add to it beeswax, rosin, and white diacalon, equal parts. If a burn is of a long time standing, and discharges very much, take mutton suet before it is tried, pound it up with chalk to the consistence of salve. This cures the most inveterate old sores of the kind.

7. *The best Salve for Women's sore Breasts ever found.*

Take one pound of tobacco, one pound spikenard, half a pound cumfrey, and boil them in three quarts of chamber ley till almost dry; squeeze out the juice, add to it pitch and beeswax, and simmer it over a moderate heat to the consistence of salve. Apply it to the part affected.

8. *An ointment to supple stiff joints and shrunk sinews.*

Take half a pound hog's lard; put into it a small handful of melolet (or Melilot) green, stew it well together, strain it off, add to it one ounce rattle-snake's grease, do. of olive oil, ten drops of oil lavender, mixed well together, Oint three times a day and rub it in well with the hand.

9. *A valuable cure for inveterate old sore legs.*

Take the bark of cavron wood or shrub maple, boil it very strong, take part of the liquor and boil it down to a salve, and wash the part affected every time it is dressed. Apply new salve twice a day. Make a tea of the same, and drink three times a day.

10. *To cure the bite of a rattle snake.*

Take green hoarhound tops, pound them fine, press out the juice, let the patient drink a table spoonful of the juice, morn, noon, and night, or three times in twenty-four hours; apply the pounded herbs to the bite, change the same twice a day. The patient may drink a spoonful of sweet olive oil. This seldom fails curing.

11. *A cure for the Itch.*

Take a half a pound of hog's lard, four ounces spirits turpentine, two ounces flour sulphur, and mix them together cold; apply it to the ancles, knees, wrists, and elbows, and rub it in the palms of the hands, if there be any raw spots; apply a little three nights when going to bed.

12. *The red salve for swellings in formation.*

Take linseed oil one pound, sweet oil, or fresh butter half a pound, red lead one pound, boil them together, stir it while boiling, then slack the heat & add to it two pounds of beeswax, 1 pound rosin, and stir them together till cold.

13. *Foote's Ointment.*

Take one pound of hog's lard, one pound of mutton tallow, half a pound oil of spike, and heat them over a moderate fire until they are united, then add as much beeswax and rosin as will make it to a salve, the renowned Foote's Ointment. This cures all common sores where there is no inflammation.

14. *A certain cure for Corns on the feet or toes.*

Take white pine turpentine, spread a plaster, apply it to the corn, let it stay on till it comes off itself. Repeat this three times—never fails curing.

15. *A cure for Warts on any part of the body.*

Make a strong solution with corrosive sublimate, wet the wart three or four times a day—never fails curing.

16. *An excellent family Bilious Pill.*

This pill made frequent use of, prevents all kinds of fevers. Take one pound of sweet rind aloes, four ounces jalap, four ounces pulverized blood root, two ounces cloves, and two ounces saffron, and beat them all to a fine powder; pill them with molasses—mix them well in a mortar. The common way of using them is to take every night one, the bigness of a pea, if you have a bilious habit; but if you wish them to act as a physic, take four or five on going to bed. They give no pain in the operation.

17. *For the tooth ache, if the tooth be hollow.*

Take gum opium, gum camphor, and spirits of turpentine, equal parts, rub them in a mortar to a paste, dip lint in the paste and put it in the hollow of the tooth every time after eating. Make use of this three or four days, and it will generally cure the tooth from ever aching.

18. *For the Bilious Colic.*

Take the above mentioned bilious pill, add to it half the weight in calomel, give four or five pills and repeat the dose, and it is a certain cure for the bilious colic. Or take mandrake roots, dried and pulverized. A large tea spoonful is a dose. This must be repeated several times.

19. *A sure cure for the canker in the mouth.*

Take one pound of fresh butter, put it into an earthen vessel well glazed, set it on the fire, let it boil, when boiling add to it four common green frogs, put them in alive, let them stew until the frogs are dry, take them out, add to it a little cammomile and parsley, when cold stir in a little burnt alum, pulverized, and if the fever is high, give a little rattlesnake's gall, dried in chalk. This will cure the most inveterate canker in the mouth, throat, or stomach.

20. *A medicine to cure inward ulcers.*

Take sassafras root bark two ounces, coltsfoot root two ounces, blood root one ounce, gum myrrh one ounce, winter bark one ounce, suckatrine aloes one ounce; steep them in two quarts of spirits, and drink a small glass every morning, fasting.

21. *For cramp in the stomach, or any inward part.*

Take ten drops of the oil of lavender on sugar or in wine. Repeat the dose once in an hour if required.

22. *A cure for the flying Rheumatism.*

Take princes pine tops, horse radish roots, elecampane roots, prickly ash bark, bittersweet bark off the root, wild cherry bark, and mustard seed—a small handful of each; one gill of tar water into a pint of brandy, or the same proportion. Drink a small glass before eating, three times a day.

23. *A valuable remedy for wind colic in women and children.*

Take equal parts of ginseng and white root, half as much

calamus or angelica seeds, dry them, pound them very fine, mix them together; a tea spoonful is a dose for a grown person, for children less, according to their age. Repeat the dose once in half an hour, if required. Very rare it ever fails.

24. *For a hectic Cough.*

Take three yolks of hen's eggs, three spoonfuls of honey, and one of tar, beat them well together, add to them one gill of wine. Take a teaspoonful three times a day before eating. Or a syrup made of barley, and turnips and elecampane; boil them in fair water, three quarts to one pint of barley, one pound of turnips, four ounces of elecampane; boiled down to one pint, add to it one pound of honey or loaf sugar, and half pint of brandy. A table spoonful is a dose, three times a day. Or wild licorice half a pound, brook liverwort half a pound, elecampane two ounces, solomon's seal four ounces, spikenard half a pound, gumfire four ounces, boiled in four quarts of water to one; add to it two pounds of honey, one pint of old spirits. Half a glass is a dose before eating.

25. *For the Earisiply, or St. Anthony's Fire.*

Make egg wine rich and good for drinking; drink a part of it, and wash the affected with the other part. This is a valuable remedy.

26. *For the Rheumatism in the loins.*

The oil of sassafras, used internal and external; ten drops on loaf sugar is a dose. Oint the part affected with the same. Repeat it as often as needful.—Or set over hemlock boughs and drink poke berries in Brandy for three weeks every day. Only seat three times—Or shower with cold water, and drink brandy all the time.—Or drink brandy, and bathe the part affected with salt and rum, hot as can be borne by a fire. Repeat it six days.

27. *For the Quincy.*

Bleed under the tongue in the first stage of it, and sweat the throat and neck with cardis, a thorny herb growing in gardens. Boil it in milk and water, and sweat powerfully three or four times. This has not failed in one instance to cure.

28. *A remarkable Plaster to ease the pain of felons, or frog felons, or any such tumour on the hands or feet, or elsewhere.*

Get a pitch pine knot from an old log, the side next to or in the ground; split the knot fine, boil out half a pound of pitch; take four ounces of strong tobacco, boil it in water, strain out the tobacco, boil the liquor until it is thick, then add the pitch to the liquor, simmer it over a moderate heat, stir it all the time till it form a salve altogether. If the swelling be on the hand or finger, lay the plaster on the wrist, if on the foot or toe, lay the plaster on the ancle; or wherever it may be, lay it above the next joint. This will take out all the pain in a short time. Dress the sore with any other salve that is best. This cure is infallible.

29. *For the Phthisic.*

Take four ounces of hen's fat and a seed bowl of skunk cabbage that grows at the bottom of the leaves close to the ground, cut it fine, stew it in the fat till it is dry, strain it off. A tea spoonful is a dose to take three times a day. Make a syrup of white swamp honeysuckle blossoms and queen of the meadow roots, sweetened with honey; add to a quart of the syrup, half a pint of brandy.

30. *To cure a Wen.*

Take clean linen rags and burn them on a pewter dish, and gather the oil on the pewter with lint, cover the wen with it twice a day. Continue it for some time, and the wen will drop out without any further trouble.

31. *An excellent remedy for the Asthma.*

Take spikenard root two ounces, sweet flag root two ounces, elecampane root two ounces, common chalk two ounces, beat very fine in a mortar, add to it a pound of honey, and beat it well together. A tea spoonful is a dose three times a day.

32. *An excellent Pill for the Hystericks.*

Take a quantity of white root, otherwise called Canada root, boil it in fair water, when it is boiled very soft, strain out the roots, and boil the liquor to the consistence of a thick paste, so that it may be pilled. Let the patient take two or three pills at a dose when the disorder is coming on.

33. *A cure for bleeding at the stomach.*

Take a pound of yellow dock root, dry it thoroughly, pound it fine, boil it in a quart of sweet milk; strain it off, drink a gill three times a day. Take also a pill of white pine turpentine every day to heal the vessels that leak.

34. *For the Dropsy.*

Take half a pound of blue flag root, half a pound of elecampane root, boiled in two gallons of fair water to one quart, sweetened with one pint of molasses. Let the patient take half a gill three times a day before eating.

35. *For the Canker Rash.*

White birch root pulverized very fine, given in small doses three or four times a day. Make a tea of the same for constant drink. For the fever give rattle snake's gall, three grains at a time.

36. *For any Hemorrhage of the Blood.*

Take a handful of blood weed—it grows in old fields, and is called by some, horse tail, or white top—is about waist or shoulder high, one stalk from the bottom, and has a very bushy top;—when it is green, pound it, and press out the juice, and give the patient a table spoonful at a time, once an hour till it stops; if it be dry boil it strong, and give the tea, very strong, three or four spoonfuls at a time.

37. *A cure for the Gravel in the Bladder or Kidneys.*

Make a strong tea of the herb called heart's ease, drink plenty.—Or take the root of Jacob's ladder, and make a very strong tea, and drink plenty. It is a most certain remedy.—Jacob's ladder is a vine that grows often in rich interval soil, near a wood or bush that stands near grass land. It comes up with one stalk about breast high, then springs off into a number of branches covered with green leaves, and the fruit is a large bunch of black berries, when ripe the bunch hangs down under the leaves by a small stem. This is proved to be the best cure that has been found.

38. *A valuable remedy for the Piles*

If the piles are outward, make an ointment of cammomile, sage, parsley, and burdoc, the leaves of each—simmer them in fresh butter or hog's lard and sweet oil. Anoint the parts with it, and drink tar water, half a gill three times a day.—But if they are inward, or blind piles, drink tar water twice a day, and essence of fir every night going to bed, half a small glass. This effects a cure in about two months.

39. *For the tooth ache, if the tooth be hollow.*

Put into the hollow a piece of blue vitrol, as much as the hollow will contain. Repeat it for several days and it will kill the marrow.

40. *For the common Canker in children or adults.*

Take canker root, or cold water root, so called, because used with cold water; wash the root, pound it, steep it in cold water, wash the tumour with the water, and drink of it. This root grows in rich soil, in meadows, by fences, stumps, or log-heaps. It comes up with a stalk from the ground a yard or two high and then branches out very large. Its leaf is like clover. The top of the root is yellow as gold, in a bunch, then branches out into many fibres, some like plantain.

41. *For the Hooping Cough.*

A syrup made of elecampane root and honey, four ounces of the root to half a pint of honey. Bake it in a well glazed earthen pot in an oven half hot. If the root be green, it needs no water; if dry, add half a pint of water. A tea spoonful of the syrup for a small child, add a little if older, three times a day.

42. *For Rickets in Children—in the bowels.*

One ounce of Rhubarb powdered in one ounce of Enceviniris, put into one quart of wine or brandy.—If the child is a year old, it may take a table spoonful at a time, if older take more, to half a gill for an adult. If any part of the body is affected with the disorder, bathe the part with brandy, and drink turkey-root steeped in wine three or four times a day.

43. *A sure remedy for women's sore nipples.*

When the infant stops sucking, apply a plaster of balsam fir. It will cure in three or four days.

44. *A cure for itching heels or feet, or ribbed heels.*

Take any kind of tallow and tallow the part affected with it, and rub it in by a hot fire at night going to bed. Repeat it three or four times.

45. *A preservative against all sorts of bilious fevers.*

The fulness of bile is the cause of all sorts of fevers, and jaundice, and bilious colic, and cholera morbus. Physic often with blood root and mandrake roots mixed together, once a quarter, and make small beer with elder roots, spruce boughs, burdock roots, hops, white ash bark, sarsaparilla roots and spikenard. Make a bitter with unicorn roots and bark, of white wood roots and the yellow dust of hops. If a family will continue this method they will never be troubled with fevers.

46. *For convulsion Fits.*

Take convulsion roots, make a tea of them and drink, or powder them and take the powder in small doses.—Convulsion root grows in timber land, and comes up in July, with a bunch of white stalks about six or eight inches high, with a little knob on the top. It has no leaves. The top and root are for use. The root is a bunch of small fibres, very numerous, and full of little knobs about the size of mustard seed, and they grow just under the leaves.

47. *For the Consumption.*

Take half a bushel of barley malt, put it into a large tub, take six pails of water, make it boil, pour it on to the malt, let it stand six hours, take half a bushel of white pine bark, one pound spikenard root, one pound Syria grass, boil them in the water that the malt is soaked in, half away, then put it into a keg, add yeast or emptins to it, let it ferment, then bottle it up, and drink one pint a day.

48. *For the Quinsy in the throat.*

Sweat the throat with spotted cardis boiled in milk and water, by holding a pot of it under the throat as hot as can be borne, and hold some of it in the mouth, and when the swelling is gone down, wear a piece of black silk about the neck constantly, and it will prevent quinsy from coming again.

49. *For swellings that come of themselves.*

An ointment made of alder tags and sugar of lead, simmered in hog's lard, and melilot and saffron, simmered all together. Strain off, and anoint the part affected, it will scatter the swelling if taken in time. Give the patient something to guard the stomach before ointing.

50. *An excellent poultice for old inveterate sores.*

Scrape yellow carrots, wilt them on a pan or fire Shovel, very soft. It takes out the inflammation and the swelling, and is an excellent poultice for a sceris breast.

51. *An excellent medicine for inward hurts or ulcers.*

Take elecampane, cumfrey, spikenard, masterwort, angelica, and ginseng roots, of each a pound, boughs of fir two pounds, cammomile one pound; put them into a still, with a gallon of rum, and two gallons of water, draw off six quarts, drink a small glass night and morning.

52. *Another excellent essence, good for all sorts of inward weakness, inward fevers, coughs, or pain in the side, stomach or breast.*

Take twenty pounds of fir boughs, one pound of spikenard, four pounds of red clover, put them into a still with ten gallons of cider, draw off three gallons, drink half a gill night and morning.

53. *For the Diabetes.*

Take a weather sheep's bladder, put it into a glass bottle that will hold a quart, fill it up with good Madeira wine, and let it stand forty-eight hours, then drink three or four times a day, about half a gill at a time. A deer's bladder is preferable.

54. *For stoppage of water.*

Take a spoonful of honey bees, as much buds of currant bushes, steep them in hot water very strong, drink two spoonfuls at a time every half hour.

55. *For sore eyes.*

White vitriol one tea spoonful, sugar of lead one do. gun powder two do. to one quart of fair water, mixed and shook well together, six or eight times. Wash the eyes three times a day—an infallible cure.

56. *For the Dropsy.*

Sassafras bark of the root one pound, prickly ash bark one pound, spice wood bush half a pound, three ounces of garlics, four ounces of parsley roots, four ounces of horse radish roots, four ounces of black birch bark—boil all in three gallons of malt beer. Drink a gill three times a day.

57. *To stop a fever sore from coming to a head, and carry it away.*

Sweat it with flannel cloths dipt in hot brine. The cloths must be changed as often as they are cold, for three hours, then wash it in brandy and wrap it in flannel; repeat it three or four times.

58. *To stop puking.*

Take gum camphor, pound it, pour on boiling water, let the patient drink a spoonful every ten minutes. It must be sweetened with loaf sugar. Or take a handful of green wheat, or grass, pound it, pour a little water on it, press out the juice, and let the patient drink a spoonful once in ten minutes.

59. *For the Lock Jaw.*

When any person is taken with the lock jaw, give him five grains of Dover's powders, then set him in a tub of hot water, as hot as he can bear it, bathe his head with camphorated spirits, let him sit or stand in the water as long as he can bear it without fainting, and bleed him if possible. Repeat this three or four times; when out of the water put him in a warm bed, wrapped in flannel.

60. *For the Numb Palsy.*

When a person is taken with the numb palsy, let blood freely if possible, give a table spoonful of flour of sulphur once an hour, bathe the part affected with spirits of hartshorn, take one pound of roll brimstone, boil it in four quarts of water to one quart, let the patient drink a table spoonful once an hour. If applied early, will finally carry it off.

B

61. *To cure vegetable poison, running ivy, or poison elder, or any other.*

Take rosemary leaves or blossoms, make a tea of it to drink morn and night, like bohea tea or any other. Or, take wild turnips, if green pound them and press out the juice, if dry boil them in fair water, wash the part affected with the clear liquor. Take part of the liquor, add to it a little saffron and camphor, and drink to cleanse the fluids and guard the stomach.

62. *For the spinevantosey that comes in the breast.*

Take spikenard root, comfrey root, yellow oak bark, tobacco, boil them in water, strong, take out some of the liquor to wash the tumour, add to the rest hog's lard or mutton tallow, beeswax and rosin, simmer it over a slow fire, stir it constantly until it is salve, apply it to the sore, physic with mandrake roots three or four times. Bleed once.

63. *To cure inward Ulcers.*

Sassafras root bark two ounces, coltsfoot root two ounces, bloodroot two ounces, gum myrrh one ounce, steeped in two quarts of spirits. Drink a small glass every morning. Live on simple diet as much as possible. For constant drink, make a beer of barley malt, one peck, spikenard root two pounds, comfrey root one pound, burdock roots two pounds, black spruce boughs five pounds, angelica root one pound, fennel seed four ounces, for ten gallons of beer. Drink one quart a day. Let your exercise be light.

64 *For the catarrh in the head.*

Take yellow dock root, split it and dry it in an oven, blood root and scoke root, four ounces of each, cinnamon one ounce, cloves half an ounce, pound them very fine, let the patient use it as snuff eight or ten times a day. Every night smoke a pipe full of cinnamon mixed with a little tobacco, and sweat the head with hemlock, brandy and camphor. Pour a little comphorated spirits and brandy into the hot liquor to sweat.

65. *For an inflammation in the head.*

Take red beets, pound them very fine, press out some of the juice, let the patient snuff some up into the head, and make a poultice of the beets, and lay it on the mould of the head. For the fever, use rattle snake's gall, cream tartar, and head bitney. Bleed as often as once a day. Physic with deerweed root, or wild mandrake roots, with a little bloodroot. Keep strong drafts to the feet.

66. *To take a film from a person's eye.*

Take sugar of lead, make it very fine, take an oat straw, cut it short, so as to be hollow through, dip the end of the straw in the powder, and blow a little of it into the film morning and night. After the film is almost consumed, apply to it a drop of hen's fat once a day until it is well.

67. *To cure a breach or burst on the body.*

Take four or five snails that crawl about on old rotten wood; you may often find them under loose bark that is moist, or on old logs or stumps. Collect a parcel of them, enough to cover the breach, lay them on a linen cloth, bind them on, and repeat it as often as the snails are dry. Let the patient drink Turkey root, cinnamon, cloves and maize, made in a tea or steeped in wine, three or four times a day. This well attended to will perform a cure.

68. *To cure a scirrhous jaw, or swelled face, or the scurvy in the mouth or teeth.*

Take prince pine and scurvy grass; boil them in water, add to it rum and honey, hold it in the mouth as hot as it can be borne, and boil a large quantity of the herbs, and sweat the head over it.

69. *A receipt to make the best Turlington balsam.*

This balsam of life is a most excellent medicine in consumptive complaints, and also for weakly females in all stages of life. For a fevery stomach let the patient take 13 or 14 drops in a small glass of wine in the morning, fasting. It strengthens the stomach, and kills the fever. It is good for pain in the stomach or side, and nourishes weak lungs, and helps a small hooping cough. This Balsam of Life is made thus: Gum Benzoin 4 ounces, Gum Storax Calhmtee 3 ounces, Balsam Telue 1 ounce, Gum Aloes Sucatine 1 1-2 ounce, Gum Albanum 1 1-2 ounce, Gum Myrrth 1 1-2 ounce, root of Angelica 2 ounces, tops of Johnswort 2 ounces. Pound all these together, put them into three pints of rectified spirits of wine in a glass bottle, let them stand in the spirits four weeks in a moderate heat, shake them once a day, strain it off, it is fit for use; and if the gums are not all dissolved, add a little more spirits to the same, shake it, and let it stand as before.

70. *For a relaxation of the gut or fundament in children.*

Break two or three hen's eggs, part the white from the yolk, take the yolks and put them into a fryingpan washed clean from grease, set them over a slow fire, let them stand a while, then turn them over and squeeze them until the oil comes out. Be careful not to burn them. Collect the oil, anoint the gut when it is down, then boil an egg very hard, let it be whole and whilst it is warm wrap it in a linen cloth, and bind it on the fundament after you have put up the gut.

71. *For the common phthisic in children.*

Take four ounces of sinical snake root, four ounces of spikenard, four ounces of parsley root, liquorice stick two ounces; boil them altogether in four quarts of water—strain off, sweeten with loaf sugar or honey, let the patient drink a small glass night and morning.

72. *For a shrunk sinew, or a stiff joint.*

Half an ounce of yellow besilicom, half an ounce of green melilot, half an ounce of oil amber, a piece of blue vitrol as big as a chesnut, simmer them together to a salve or ointment, apply it to the part affected, and on the joint above. Repeat it often and it will perform the cure.

73. *For the Rheumatism.*

Take a handful of prince of pine, a handful of horse radish roots, elecampane roots, prickly ash bark, bittersweet root bark, wild cherry bark, mustard seed, and a pint of tar water put into two quarts of brandy. Drink a small glass every morning, noon and night, before eating. Bathe the part affected with salt and rum, by a warm fire.

74. *A remedy for weakness in the urine vessels, for children that cannot hold their water.*

For those so troubled, take good red bark two ounces, one quart of wine, steep the bark in the wine 24 hours; let the patient drink a table spoonful if two or three years old, if older, a little more at a time. Or, red beech bark, taken off a green tree, dry it well, pulverize it fine, and use the same way.

75. *For the nose bleed.*

Take the common nettleroots, dry them and carry them in the pocket, and chew them every day. Continue this three weeks.

76. *To cure a consumptive cough or pain in the breast.*

Take a spoonful of common tar, three spoonfuls of honey, three yolks of hen's eggs, and half a pint of wine; beat the tar, eggs and honey well together, then add the wine, and beat all well together in a dish, with a knife or spoon. Bottle it up fit for use. A tea spoonful is a dose, morning, noon, and night, before eating. Drink barley tea for constant drink.

77. *For weakly obstructions in the female sex.*

Take hearts ease herbs, spikenard roots, with the pith out, a small part of blood root, turkey root, wild liquorice, a few roots of white pond lilies, a good parcel of female flowers, so called. It often grows by the sides of ponds, and has a leaf and blossom some like cowslips—but it grows single, one root or stalk by itself, and some smaller than the cowslip; the leaves are green, and the blossom is yellow. This is one of the finest of roots for the female use in the world. Take double the quantity of this, and equal parts of the others, make a syrup of them; boil them in fair water until all the substance is out, strain it off, sweeten it with honey, add as much rum to it as will keep it from souring. Drink half a gill going to bed every night. This will strengthen the system, and throw off all obstructions. It is best for any person so complaining, to wear a thick piece of flannel on the small of the back.

78. *For children troubled with worms.*

There are many things helpful to children troubled with

worms. The bark of witch hazel, or spotted alder, steep it in a pewter vessel, let it boil, on a moderate heat very strong; a child of a year old can take a table spoonful, if older, take more, according to the age. Let them take it four or five times in a day for several days. It is sure and safe.—Or take sage, powder it fine, mix it with honey; a tea spoonful is a dose.—Sweetened milk, with a little alum added to it is very good to turn worms.—Flour sulphur mixed with honey, is very good for worms.—Take a piece of steel, heat it very hot in a smith's fire, then lay on it a roll of brimstone, melt the steel, let it fall off into water, it will be in round lumps; take them and pound them very fine, mix the dust with molasses; let the child take half a tea spoonful night and morning, fasting.—Wild mandrake roots dried and powdered mixed with honey; give a child of a year old as much of the powder as will lie on sixpence; take it in the morning fasting, three or four times successively.—If a child is taken with fits by reason of worms, give as much paregorick as the child can bear. It will turn the worms and ease the child.—To prevent children from having worms, let them eat onions raw or cooked, raw is best.—Salt and water is good to turn worms, and give a dose or two of flour sulphur, mixt with molasses or honey, after; brings off the worms without any thing else.

79. *A cure for the Polypus.*

Take two ounces of bloodroot, dry it, pound it fine, quarter of an ounce of calix cinnamon, two ounces of scokeroot, snuff it up the nose, it will kill the polypus. Then take a pair of forceps and pull it out, and use the snuff until it is cured. If the nose is so stopped that it cannot be snuffed up, boil the same and gurgle it in the throat, and sweat the head with the hot liquor until it withers so as to use the snuff.

80. *For a frog under the tongue.*

When the frog is first perceived, take weak ley and hold it in the mouth as hot as can be borne, and if it is grown tough, touch it in three or four places with caustic until it is sore, then apply the ley.

81. *For Childbed fevers.*

In childbed fevers take rattle snake's gall, five grains malitel, sweet balm tea once an hour until the fever abates, and every time the fever rises continue the same. Keep the body loose.

82. *Cure for phthisic.*

Roast three egg shells brown—pulverize rather coarsly; mix with half a pint of molasses and take a spoonful morning, noon, and night. The cure is certain, unless the disease is hereditary, descending from the parents.

83. *For the Dysentery.*

Half an ounce of promegranate bark, pulverised, and steeped in a pint of wine, or good cider, and taken a gill at a time, before eating.

84. *A valuable remedy for the Dysentery and bloody Flux.*

Take of white pine bark after the ross is off, three pints, of water three pints; let it simmer down to one quart; strain it off; add half a pint of West India rum, half a pint, of West India molasses; the whole composition for a grown person; half for a child.

This remedy is simple, but may be depended on as effectual: it will seldom if ever fail.

85. *To destroy worms in a safe and sure way.*

Take a large tea spoonful of the rust of tin; mix it with a table spoonful of molasses. This is a valuable remedy, it may be given in sickness or health.

PROPERTIES AND USES OF VEGETABLES.

I would wish to give the true nature of all sorts of vegetables that I have mentioned in the foregoing work.

CATNIP is a warm herb, of a diaphoretic or sweating nature.

PENNEROYAL is much the same only more powerful. It retains a very powerful pungent oil.

SPEARMINT is pungent and hot, but is of an astringent nature.

CALAMINT is much the same but not so strong.

HOARHOUND is very strengthening to the lungs, and is somewhat of a pectoral. It is excellent in a cough or stoppage in the stomach.

EVERLASTING, or Indian poesy, is a very balsamic herb, is very healing and cooling, and excellent in salves or ointments.

JOHNSWORT is much the same.

PEA BALM is a cooling, sweating herb, and is good in fevers and inflammations.

CAMMOMILE is a great restorative to the lungs, and promotes perspiration; it is good in salves and ointments to take away swellings.

MAY WEED is of a pectoral nature, and is good for a pain in the side.

GARDEN COLTSFOOT is a great restorative to the lungs, and is good in syrups for coughs.

MELILOT is good in salves and ointments for swellings and inflammations. It is mollifying and cooling.

SAGE is the greatest restorative to human nature of any herb that grows.

PARSLEY is very cooling and softening.

BLOODROOT is a powerful puke or purge; steeped in spirits it will serve for a puke, and boiled in fair water it serves as a purge.

WILD JENTON is a strong purge boiled.

MANDRAKE ROOTS are an excellent physic dried and pounded.

CUMFREY and spikenard are so well known that they need no describing.

ELECAMPANE is good in coughs, yet it is an astringent.

CRANESBILL is an astringent, and excellent in Cankers.

WHITEROOT is of a physical nature and is good to remove wind pent in the stomach, or part of the bowels.

SASSAFRAS root is good for the blood.—Likewise Sarsaparilla, Horse Radish, Burdock root, Elder roots, Hop roots, and wild Coltsfoot, are a good pectoral.

WHITE Pond Lily roots, and Yellow Lily roots the same.

FEVER BUSH. This vegetable is used by the Indians with success in all cases of inflammation.

BUTTER NUT. The bark of this tree, rightly prepared, constitutes one of the best and safest physics ever known.

WINTER'S BARK. This is the product of one of the largest trees on Terra del Fuego. It is good in dropsy and in scurvy.

CONTENTS.

1. For the King's Evil.
2. Best remedy for rattles in children.
3. Valuable remedy for the bilious colic.
4. For a Felon.
5. For the salt Rheum.
6. Salve for a Burn.
7. The best salve for Women's sore Breasts ever found.
8. An ointment to supple Stiff Joints and Shrunk Sinews.
9. An infallible cure for inveterate old sore legs.
10. To cure the bite of a rattle Snake.
11. An infallible cure for the Itch.
12. A red Salve for swellings in formation.
13. Foot's Ointment.
14. A certain cure for Corns on the feet or toes.
15. A cure for warts on any part of the body.
16. An excellent family Bilious Pill.
17. For the tooth ache, if the tooth be hollow.
18. For the Bilious Colic.
19. A sure cure for the Canker in the mouth.
20. A medicine to cure inward ulcers.
21. For the cramp in the stomach or any inward part.
22. A cure for the flying Rheumatism.
23. An infallible remedy for Wind Colic in Women and Children.
24. For a hectic Cough.
25. For the Earisiply, or St Anthony's Fire.
26. For the Rheumatism in the Loins.
27. For the Quincy.
28. A remarkable plaster to ease the pain of Felons, or Frog Felons, or any such Tumor on the Hands or feet, or elsewhere.
29. For the Phthisic.
30. To cure a Wen.
31. An excellent remedy for the Asthma.

32. An excellent pill for the Hystericks.
33. An infallible cure for bleeding at the stomach.
34. For the Dropsy.
35. For the Canker Rash.
36. For any hemorrage of the Blood.
37. A cure for the gravel in the Bladder or Kidneys.
38. An infallible cure for the piles.
39. For the Tooth Ache if the Tooth be hollow.
40. For the common Canker in Children or adults.
41. For the Hooping-Cough.
42. For Rickets in children—in the bowels.
43. A sure remedy for Women's sore Nipples.
44. A cure for itching heels or feet, or ribbed heels.
45. A preservative against all sorts of Bilious fevers.
46. For Convulsion Fits.
47. For the Consumption.
48. For the Quincy in the throat.
49. For swellings that come of themselves.
50. An excellent Poultice for old inveterate sores.
51. An excellent medicine for inward hurts or ulcers.
52. Another excellent essence, good for all sorts of inward weakness, inward fevers, coughs, or pain in the side, stomach, or breast.
53. For the Diabetes.
54. For stoppage of water.
55. For sore Eyes.
56. For the Dropsy.
57. To stop a Fever Sore from coming to a head, and carry it away.
58. To stop Puking.
59. For the Lock Jaw.
60. For the Numb Palsy.
61. To cure vegetable Poison, running Ivy, or poison Elder, or any other.
62. For the Spinevantosey that comes in the breast.
93. To cure inward Ulcers.
64. For a Catarrh in the head.
65. For an inflammation in the head.
66. To take a film from a person's Eye.
67. To cure a breach or Burst on the Body.
68. To cure a Schirrous Jaw, or swelled face, or the scurvy in the mouth or teeth.
69. A recipe to make the best Turlington Balsam.
70. For a relaxation of the fundament or gut in children.
71. For the common phthisic in children.

72. For a shrunk Sinew or Stiff Joint.
73. For the Rheumatism.
74. A remedy for weakness in the Urine vessels, for children that cannot hold their water.
75. For the Nose Bleed.
76. To cure a consumptive cough, or pain in the Breast.
77. For weakly obstructions in the Female sex.
78. For children troubled with Worms.
79. A cure for the Polypus.
80. For a Frog under the tongue.
81. For Childbed Fevers.
82. Cure for the Phthisick.
83. For the Dysentery.
84. For Dysentery and Bloody Flux.
85. To destroy worms in children.

Mr

Nort. Alice Drew
Barrington
N.H.
1830

"Mr. Thr. J. Drew

Barrington
NH
1836

www.ingramcontent.com/pod-product-compliance
Lightning Source LLC
Chambersburg PA
CBHW072044290426
44110CB00014B/1570